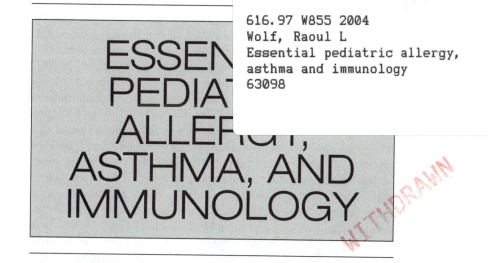

ESSENTIAL PEDIATRIC ALLERGY, ASTHMA, AND IMMUNOLOGY

NOTICE

Medicine is an ever-changing science. As new research and clinical experience broaden our knowledge, changes in treatment and drug therapy are required. The authors and the publisher of this work have checked with sources believed to be reliable in their efforts to provide information that is complete and generally in accord with the standards accepted at the time of publication. However, in view of the possibility of human error or changes in medical sciences, neither the authors nor the publisher nor any other party who has been involved in the preparation or publication of this work warrants that the information contained herein is in every respect accurate or complete, and they disclaim all responsibility for any errors or omissions or for the results obtained from use of the information contained in this work. Readers are encouraged to confirm the information contained herein with other sources. For example and in particular, readers are advised to check the product information sheet included in the package of each drug they plan to administer to be certain that the information contained in this work is accurate and that changes have not been made in the recommended dose or in the contraindications for administration. This recommendation is of particular importance in connection with new or infrequently used drugs.

ESSENTIAL PEDIATRIC ALLERGY, ASTHMA, AND IMMUNOLOGY

Raoul L. Wolf, MD

Director, Division of Pediatric Allergy, Asthma, and Immunology
University of Chicago Children's Hospital/La Rabida Children's Hospital
Professor of Pediatrics
University of Chicago School of Medicine
Chicago, Illinois

McGraw-Hill
MEDICAL PUBLISHING DIVISION

New York / Chicago / San Francisco / Lisbon / London
Madrid / Mexico City / Milan / New Delhi / San Juan
Seoul / Singapore / Sydney / Toronto

Essential Pediatric Allergy, Asthma, and Immunology

1 2 3 4 5 6 7 8 9 0   DOC/DOC 0 9 8 7 6 5 4

ISBN 0-07-141668-4

This book was set in Times Roman by International Typesetting and Composition.
The editor was James Shanahan.
The editorial assistant was Marta Victoria Colon.
The production supervisor was Richard Ruzycka.
Project management was provided by International Typesetting and Composition.
RR Donnelley was printer and binder.
This book was printed on acid-free paper.

Library of Congress Cataloging-in-Publication Data

Essential pediatric allergy, asthma and immunology / edited by Raoul Wolf.–1st ed.
    p. ; cm.
  Includes bibliographical references.
  ISBN 0-07-141668-4
  1. Immunologic diseases in children. 2. Allergy in children. 3. Asthma in children. I. Wolf, Raoul.
  [DNLM: 1. Hypersensitivity–diagnosis–Child. 2. Hypersensitivity–diagnosis–Infant. 3. Hypersensitivity–therapy–Child. 4. Hypersensitivity–therapy–Infant. 5. Immunologic Diseases–diagnosis–Child. 6. Immunologic Diseases–diagnosis–Infant. 7. Immunologic Diseases–therapy–Child. 8. Immunologic Diseases–therapy–Infant. WD 300 E787 2004]
RJ385.E87 2004
618.92'97–dc22
                                        2004042649

To Gill, Saul, Isa-Lee, and Knight

CONTENTS

PREFACE

What is really the nature of allergy? We tend to think of such knowledge as a purely twentieth century development. Yet the concepts of allergy, represented by symptoms like bloating, itching, dizziness, or headache were documented more than 2000 years ago, by the Greek physician Hippocrates.

Asthma, too, is not as recent an arrival on the research scene as we may believe. As long ago as the twelfth century, a sufferer named Prince Al-Afdal sought treatment from the physician to the Court of Saladin. Even today, the regimen this doctor prescribed seems sensible. He recommended self-control with food and drink, avoidance of any polluted city environment, and moderate enjoyment of that ageless comfort food—chicken soup. Included in the list of treatments were inhalations made from strophanthin leaves, now known to contain a high concentration of atropine. This drug and other anticholinergics are still useful for acute asthma. The physician concerned was the distinguished Moses Maimonides, who died in 1204, but whose treatise on the subject, *On Asthma*, is still in print.

Maimonides' practical advice notwithstanding, there was little understanding of these immunologic problems until Cooper, Peterson, and Good, working with chickens, provided the first clear description of the origin of the two essential subcategories of lymphocytes, T cells and B cells. Since then, our knowledge of immunology and allergy has expanded exponentially with increasing understanding of the details of its intricate response and control mechanisms. With this knowledge, however, we have realized how little of the immune system is truly understood.

We now know that immune function is extremely complicated, and that its workings are not easy to interpret. This book is an attempt to make this complex topic more accessible without reducing it to an oversimplified framework. For this reason, the book is divided into three sections: basic allergy and immunology, clinical features, and diagnosis and treatment.

The first chapter describes the function of the immune system and leads the reader into its more complex aspects. Within the context of immune function, the opening chapter also discusses the development of immune components during embryogenesis in a way that eases understanding of recurrent infections and immune defects, both of which are examined in detail in later chapters of the book.

The next topic, development of allergy, presents the unique mechanisms involved in allergic reactions and discusses the four basic types of immune injury. There are cogent examples of each. Type I immune injury is the result of the action of IgE on mast cells, Type II is mediated by IgG which causes direct damage to normal cell components, Type III is also caused by IgG which forms circulating immune complexes that produce vasculitis and cell damage, and Type IV is the result of the interaction of T cells and macrophages and does not require immunoglobulin.

Also discussed is the hygiene hypothesis, at whose heart lies the statement that asthma and allergies begin in childhood or even infancy, irrespective of when they present clinically. Its prominence as an important shift in the paradigm of early development of allergic disorders has given this hypothesis a pivotal place in both favorable and oppositional research, so it merits a chapter to itself.

Chapter Four and following deal with clinical presentation that helps determine and guide the therapy of allergic and immunologic disorders. Common allergic skin disorders, atopic dermatitis, urticaria, and angioedema appear here.

Asthma is reviewed on its own, since it involves many individual issues, such as the rise in frequency and morbidity of asthma among children and young teenagers. Case studies, discussions of new concepts in pathophysiology, and remarks on the role of guidelines from the National Institutes of Health subsidiary, the National Heart, Lung, and Blood Institute, are all aimed at easing the challenges of assessing and managing such patients.

The diagnosis and management of the wheezing infant is reviewed only briefly in the chapter on asthma but at greater length in a chapter on its own. This is because it is a difficult and pressing problem, and well worth the chapter assigned solely to its discussion. There is an extensive differential diagnosis for this condition, which is addressed in this chapter.

Likewise assigned to a chapter on its own is allergic rhinitis, which, inexplicably, is one of medicine's most underrated ailments. As compared with a control group, patients with this distressing condition have a noticeably lower quality of life in multiple domains; yet the condition is often taken less seriously than it deserves. Here, the reader will find an in-depth review of its causes, presentation, differential diagnosis, and management, as well as a discussion of the complications which underlie its potential severity.

From clinical presentation, the book turns next to investigation and interpretation, the discussion resting on an important fact—that the investigation of allergies is often equally frustrating for physician and patient. The chapter on Investigation of Allergies presents an approach to solve a frequently-encountered dilemma; what is causing the allergic reaction? The keys to detection of a cause lie in obtaining a careful history and in the judicious use of allergy investigations. Pulmonary function studies are probably underused in children, but are as useful in these patients as they are in adults. The methods and interpretation of these studies are presented in their own chapter from a practical clinical viewpoint, with examples provided by clinical scenarios

Detection of immune defects is a two-part process. The chapter "Immune Deficiency and Recurrent Infections" details the two-stage investigation. The first is a screening battery of tests that includes a complete blood count and differential, quantitative immunoglobulins and an assessment of specific antibody production. The second stage, used if the first is abnormal or suspicious, is highly specialized and includes evaluations of T-cell and B-cell function and surface markers. Some centers can measure specific cell receptors and mediators. Both first- and second-stage investigations are explained in the chapter, with guidelines for use and interpretation of the tests.

The final chapters focus on treatment. This essential aspect of management appears in the chapter "Medications and Therapeutic Methods," where drug doses and delivery systems are presented in detail. This chapter will serve well for just finding a drug dose or for a detailed consideration of the approach to treating a specific disease. Finally, the closing chapters examine two significant, but often overlooked approaches to the management of allergies. These are environmental control and allergy immunotherapy.

ACKNOWLEDGMENT

I thank James Shanahan, my editor, for his excellent suggestions and comments on the design of this book and encouragement throughout this challenging project.

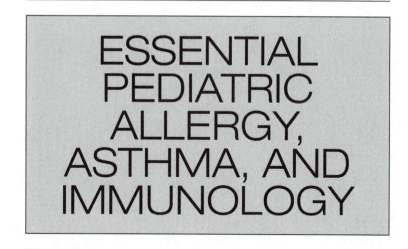

ESSENTIAL
PEDIATRIC
ALLERGY,
ASTHMA, AND
IMMUNOLOGY

1

FUNCTION AND DEVELOPMENT OF THE IMMUNE SYSTEM IN HUMANS

PURPOSE OF THE IMMUNE SYSTEM

Immune function has evolved continuously since the earliest nematodes. By this process, it has become the most complex and essential system in the body. In this chapter, we review the function of this complex system, and review this function in the context of embryologic development. The key to understanding immune deficiencies lies in the embryology of the immune system. Over time, the steps of an immune reaction have come to consist of a series of highly integrated operations, each with delicate feedback control mechanisms. Few cells in the body are not involved in one way or another in an immunological response, but the cells that primarily regulate the immune response are of the mononuclear series.

Essentially, the primary function of the immune system is eliminating potentially dangerous proteins and other substances foreign to the body. Such a substance is described as an antigen, whatever its origin. An antigen is thus defined as any compound that will provoke an immune response.

Among the most significant antigens are invading microbes and other disease causing organisms. Equally important are potentially cancerous cells as they emerge in the body. These antigens are removed by activated immunologic cells and their products, the most important of which are antibodies. There is thus a twofold response of cellular mechanisms and soluble proteins. This combination of a direct and an indirect defense provides sufficient capacity to destroy any antigen or antigens that the body may encounter.

In addition, the effects of immunological regulation are widespread throughout the body and may have a significant impact on many other organs. For example, researchers have recently found a complex interaction between the function of the immune and the central nervous systems. It has also been noted that the growth of several blood cells depends on factors released by mononuclear cells. Moreover, there is a close interplay between blood clotting mechanisms and the complement proteins of the immune system. The function of many other organs may also be affected by the panoply of substances released by the cells of the immune system.

The development of the immune system and its complex interactions begins early in fetal life and continues maturing throughout embryogenesis. At the time of birth and for several months, the immune response receives a boost when the infant is suddenly exposed to a large number of antigens. However, the child does not reach adult levels of function until after the first year of life.

FUNCTION OF THE IMMUNE SYSTEM

Components

Cells

There are two types of cells involved in the immune response, mononuclear and multinuclear.

Mononuclear Cells

This group includes lymphocytes, monocytes and macrophages. The lymphocytes are most unusual in that they have the appearance of a cell near the end of its life cycle, but are capable of reverting to a blast cell and undergoing rapid cell division. It is during this cell division that these cells control and stimulate the immune response. There are two further subgroups of lymphocytes, T cells and B cells. The T cells are the sensing (afferent) arm of the immune response and detect and respond to the presence of an antigen. B cells are the effector (efferent) arm and produce antibodies. Macrophages are the cells that initially come into contact with antigens and are responsible for "alerting" the lymphocytes of a foreign invader. They can also destroy many antigens directly. Monocytes are a circulating form of macrophages. Plasma cells are end stage cells that derive from B cells and are responsible for the secretion of antibodies into plasma.

Mast cells are not generally part of the response to antigens. They are large cells that contain granules in which are preformed histamine and eosinophil chemotactic agents. Their function is discussed in more detail in the chapter Basis of Allergy.

Multinuclear

Polymorphonuclear cells are the scavenger cells of the immune system that digest and destroy antigens, usually after they have bonded to antibodies. They are very mobile blood cells that constantly migrate in and out of tissues. The role of *eosinophils* in the usual immune response is less clear, and they are probably only involved in the control of parasites.

Humoral

There are not actually two separate components of the immune response. There is a continuum of reaction from the cellular reaction to production of antibodies. *Immunoglobulins* are proteins that include antibodies that are produced by B cells and plasma cells. They bind specifically to antigens. *Complement proteins* are actually a series of enzymes that activate each other, and produce a series of effects that include coating antigens so that they are more easily ingested by polymorphonuclear cells (PMNs). There are also many byproducts of this activation that have potent effects, such as attracting PMNs to the site of the immune response (Table 1-1).

TABLE 1-1

COMPONENTS OF THE IMMUNE SYSTEM

Cellular
Mononuclear
Lymphocytes
T cells
B cells
Monocytes
Macrophages
Multinucleate
Polymorphonuclear cells
Eosinophils
Humoral
Immunoglobulins
Complement

OVERVIEW OF IMMUNE FUNCTION

An outline of the mechanisms of immune interactions is presented in Figure 1-1. An antigen is bound to an antigen presenting cell and is presented via the major histocompatibility complex (MHC) to T lymphocytes. These cells respond by reverting to a blast cell form (no other cell line in the body does this) and undergoes rapid cell division. During this process, a large number of soluble mediators, termed cytokines and interleukins, are released into the microenvironment and serum. These mediators, in the presence of antigen, stimulate B cells. These cells also revert to a blast form and undergo cell division. During this division, there is constant feedback to the B cells, and a cell line that codes for that antigen is selected. This line divides into two cell types. The first is a plasma cell, and the second is a B cell that holds the memory of the antigen in IgD on the cell surface. Plasma cells actually secrete specific antibody into plasma; B cells retain 95% of immunoglobulin on the cell surface. The antibody binds specifically with the antigen by the Fab portion. In doing so, the complement binding site is exposed, and the complement cascade is initiated. Chemoattractant breakdown products of complement are C3a, C4a, and C5a. These molecules draw PMN and eosinophils to the site of inflammation. The PMN ingest and destroy the antigen by lysozymes and other intracellular enzymes.

The basic definition of an antigen is any substance that stimulates the immune system to produce an antibody. Antigens are mostly proteins and often are enzymes. Proteins are strongly antigenic in part because of their quaternary structure that produces three-dimensional features that present more antigenic surfaces to the immune cells. These antigenic surfaces are known as epitopes, and they can contain as few as two or three amino acids. Antibodies are proteins with a common structure consisting of two heavy and two light chains. They fall into the general category of immunoglobulins, not all of which may have antibody function.

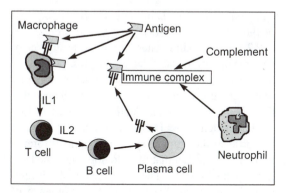

FIGURE 1-1

PATHWAY OF FUNCTION FOR AN IMMUNE RESPONSE.

An antigen is recognized as foreign by macrophages, which process the antigen. The next step is to present the antigenic material to T cells, which in turn stimulate B cells. B cells transform into plasma cells, which make a specific antibody. The antibody binds specifically to the antigen, exposing the complement binding site. Complement is activated, and some of the components attract neutrophils. These cells then ingest and destroy the antigen.

Immunoglobulin

The general structure of immunoglobulin is consistent across all antibody classes. There are two heavy chains joined to shorter light chains by disulfide bonds. There are two key segments of the immunoglobulin molecule: the *Fc* (cell) segment, which lies between the two heavy chains and the *Fab* (antibody) portion, which is found between the heavy and light chains. There are thus two Fab sites to one Fc segment. The area where the light chains join the heavy chains is known as the hinge region. This is important, as this portion of the molecule is where the complement binding site is found.

Antibodies are immunoglobulins with specifically coded Fab portion to bind selectively to an antigen. This region of the molecule is produced in response to an antigen and is termed the hypervariable region. The antigen fits between the heavy and light chains. This area of the molecule conforms to the three-dimensional map of the antigen; the affinity of the antibody for the antigen depends on how precise the fit is between these molecules. The power of the immune response lies in the ability to create a library of antibody forming cells that can produce antibodies specific for a vast array of antigens.

The Fc portion attaches to macrophages and other antigen presenting cells, polymorphonuclear cells and B cells.

The genetics of immunoglobulin production are unique. In all other circumstances, one gene produces one protein. In the case of immunoglobulins, three gene loci are involved in the production of one protein, i.e., an antibody. Two light chain loci are located on chromosomes 2 and 22, and the heavy chains are found on chromosome 14.

There are five categories of immunoglobulins (Ig). Three of these isotypes are concerned with defense immune function. These are IgG, IgM and IgA.

Defense immunoglobulins:

- IgG: Major defense against common bacteria.

There are four subclasses of IgG.

- IgM: First to increase in response to an infection.
- IgA: Main antibody in secretions.

Other functions:

- IgD: "Switch" antibody only on B-cell surface.
- IgE: Antibody causing allergies such as hay fever.

In addition, there are four subclasses of IgG.

INTEGRATION OF IMMUNE FUNCTION

Figure 1-1 shows the general response of the immune system in a sequence of activation steps. Macrophages bind and process the antigen. This information is passed on to T cells directly and via mediators known as monokines. The most important of these is interleukin 1 (IL1). T cells divide and activate B cells, which then transform into plasma cells and release specific antibody directed against the initiating antigen. This antibody then binds with the antigen, forming immune complexes and activating the complement cascade. With the release of

chemoattractants, PMNs are brought to the site and ingest and digest the complexes. Not all antigens must be processed by T cells and macrophages before B cells will respond to them. These antigens are known as *T independent antigens*.

Antibodies are produced in a specific sequence. IgM is the first produced, and is present for a short time. IgG follows, and serum levels persist for years. IgA is the last to appear, and IgA persists long term in its secretory form (Figure 1-1).

MAJOR COMPONENTS

Major Histocompatibility Complex (MHC)

MHC is the most important surface structure of the immune response and overall function of the immune system. It is present on all cells in the body and is the structure that is the molecular identity of an individual. There are two main classes of MHC, Class I and Class II.

Class I is the recognition portion of the molecule and is on all cells in the body. It is composed of three alpha units, A, B, and C and a beta unit, beta2 microglobulin. There are a large number of variants at each of the three alpha sites, giving rise to about 2×10^7 unique combinations. In other words, there is a one in twenty million chance that two people will have an identical MCH Class I by random match. Class I antigens are vital in immune response, as the immune system recognizes foreign antigens by the fact that they do not match the built in template for MHC. The development of this template is an essential aspect of the emergence of immunity in the fetus, and without it, the immune system cannot function. When an organ, such as a liver, kidney, or lung, is transplanted, the recipient and donor need to match as closely as possible at the MHC level to avoid rejection of the transplanted organ by the recipient's immune response. The function of the beta2 microglobulin portion of MHC Class I is unknown.

A Class I molecule that is not recognized by macrophages and other antigen presenting cells or

T cells will identify the MHC as foreign, and the cells will react to the foreign MHC, initiating an immune response. The Class I molecule has a further important function on macrophages, dendritic cells and Langerhans cells. It presents processed antigens, primarily viral, to CD8+ T cells and cytotoxic cells.

In experimental conditions in inbred mice, MHC identity is necessary for T cells and macrophages to interact. This restriction is not as readily seen in humans.

Class II molecules are present primarily on immune cells, and are expressed in increased density when the cells are activated. Class II molecules have a structure that is different from Class I. Class II consists of α and β chains that closely resemble the heavy and light chains of the immunoglobulin molecules and belong to a family of molecules that are similar to immunoglobulins. It is divided into HLA-DP, HLA-DQ, and HLA-DR regions. These surface structures are important in the interaction of immune active cells with each other. Class II molecules present exogenous antigens, such as bacterial products, to CD4+ cells stimulating an immune response.

The interaction of antigen presenting cells and T cells is restricted by MHC compatibility. At least in vitro, and in inbred animal models, T cells are only activated by MHC identical macrophages. In human in vitro studies, macrophages do not stimulate non-HLA identical T cells as well as autologous T cells, suggesting that there is at least a partial restriction at the MHC level in humans as well.

Cells

Macrophages

These are large cells that form the cornerstone in the regulation of the immune response. They have three main functions:

Presentation of antigen. Most antigens will attach to the surface of a macrophage. This cell then passes on information about the antigen by presenting it to T cells, activating them. This usually requires close contact between the cells, which may include temporary fusion of the outer membranes of the T cells and macrophages. The bridging molecules between the T cells and the macrophage are the structures of the MHC (Figure 1-2).

Destruction of antigen. The macrophage may ingest the antigen adhering to its surface by a process of phagocytosis. Macrophages contain the enzymes

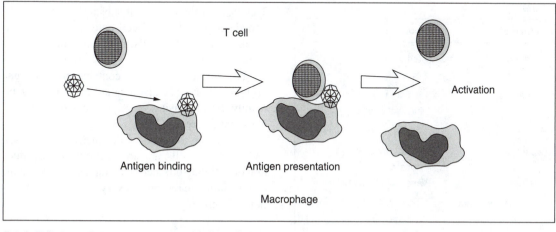

T cell

Activation

Antigen binding　　Antigen presentation

Macrophage

FIGURE 1-2

MECHANISMS OF IMMUNE INTERACTIONS.

Antigens bind to macrophage surfaces and are ingested and presented to T cells via Class I or Class II MHC resulting in the activation of both cells. Certain antigens are destroyed directly by macrophages: mycobacteria and listeria monocytogenes are common examples of this phenomenon.

necessary to digest many bacteria; these enzymes are released by the act of phagocytosis. They include lysozymes, beta glucuronidase, and lactic dehydrogenase. Some organisms, such as *Mycobacterium tuberculi* (the agent causing tuberculosis), are exclusively handled by these cells.

Initiation of the immune response. Macrophages that have been "armed" produce a large number of low molecular weight substances that have potent effects on initiating and suppressing the responses of other immune cells. These are broadly termed cytokines. The most active of these are presented in Table 1-2.

Other Antigen Presenting Cells

Cells other than macrophages can present antigen to T cells.

Langerhans cells: These are found predominantly in the skin. They may transport T cells to lymphatics.

Follicular dendritic cells: These are found in liver, spleen, and lymph nodes and interact with T and B cells. They have mainly been noted in mice.

Lymphocytes

Lymphocytes are small round cells that consist almost exclusively of a nucleus. While this is usually the appearance of a cell near the end of its life cycle, these cells are unique in that they are able to revert to a primitive form and undergo cell division. It is during this phase that they exhibit their immunological properties. There are three groups: T cells, B cells, and null cells.

There are four cellular phases to all lymphocyte responses diagramed in Figure 1-3. Binding to the surface receptors occurs in seconds, immediately followed by transduction of the signal into the cell. This signal is amplified and transmitted to receptor molecules over several hours and longer. Ultimately, these signals are translated into gene transcription during cell division, giving rise to a variety of responses.

T cells. These are very potent cells with a wide range of function. They are usually stimulated by macrophages or directly by antigen. In response, these cells divide rapidly and in doing so release a large number of soluble peptides termed lymphokines. The best described of these is interleukin 2 (IL2), which maintains the immune response of T cells. A group of several substances collectively known as polyclonal B-cell activators provides a major stimulus to B cells, initiating a broad-based response.

The surface of T cells contains protein-sugar groupings that make distinct markers. These can be readily detected using very specific antibodies and dyes that fluoresce (Table 1-3).

T cells are the primary defense against viruses and cancerous cells, and are essential for the induction of antibody production in humans, to the extent that the immune response is very poor without functional T cells.

B cells. These cells are factories for the production of antibodies. They divide in response to stimuli from T cells and produce two groups of daughter cells; one that holds memory for the antigen and will respond rapidly on reexposure, and a second that

TABLE 1-2

CYTOKINE PRODUCTION FROM MONONUCLEAR CELLS

Cytokine	Action
Interferon	Antitumor
	Antiviral
Interleukins	Mediate mononuclear cell interactions
Prostaglandins	Modulate cellular functions
Leukotrienes	Smooth muscle constriction
	Vascular permeability
Tumor necrosis factor	Induce NK cells
	Antitumor
	Antiviral
T-cell growth factor	Maintain T-cell response

Note: While these cytokines have many functions, only the most usual are listed.

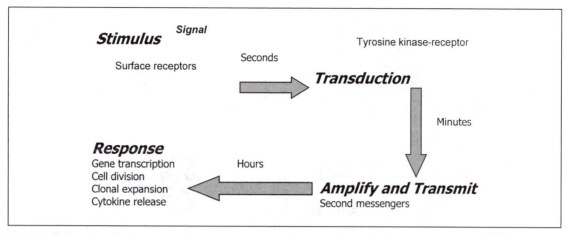

FIGURE 1-3

SIGNAL TRANSDUCTION.

There is an initial stimulus to a surface receptor, which results in transduction of that signal within seconds. Via the action of several receptors, such as tyrosine kinase, the signal is amplified via second messengers which cause nuclear effects that initiate cell division, clonal expansion, and the release of cytokines. This process takes several hours, and results in gene transcription and the formation of antibodies.

becomes a plasma cell producing large quantities of specific antibody. Plasma cells are normally found only in bone marrow, lymph nodes, and spleen (Figure 1-4).

TABLE 1-3

SURFACE MARKERS THAT DEFINE THE T-CELL SUBSETS

T-cell Subset	Function
CD3	All T cells
CD4	Helper cells
CD8	Suppressor cells
CD56	Natural killer cells
CD11	Adhesion
T receptor	All T cells
CD1a	Thymocytes

Note: CD is shorthand for cluster of differentiation. While these structures are associated with T cells that have specific function, it is an error to consider the surface marker as synonymous with the cell function. For example, CD4 cells can have helper functions, but may suppress lymphocyte function in a different study design or in vivo situation. Other CD markers function as receptors for specific chemokines.

Plasma cells. These are large cells that have a spoke wheel shaped nucleus and a very prominent Golgi apparatus and endoplasmic reticulum. They are designed to produce protein in high volume. Ninety-five percent of the antibody that is produced by plasma cells is released into blood. By contrast, B cells retain most of the immunoglobulin that they synthesize on the cell surface.

IMMUNE RECOGNITION

There are several steps in the recognition of an antigen as foreign to the host.

MHC Complex

The key to immune activation lies in the MHC complex. Macrophages and T cells scan cells for the MHC Class I antigens. If these match the template for self, the antigen will be ignored. The slightest deviation from the template for MHC stored in T-cell memory will immediately trigger an immune response. If the host MHC is altered to even a minor degree, the cell will become the target

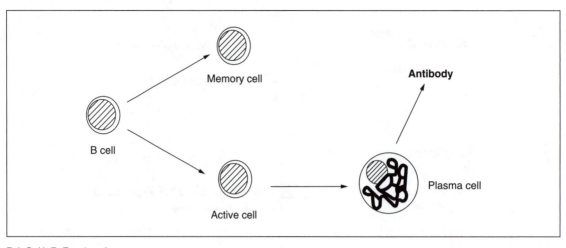

FIGURE 1-4

B CELLS.

Antigen in the presence of T cells stimulates B cells to divide. This stimulus results in the formation of two populations of B cell. One transforms into plasma cells and produces antibody, while the other becomes a memory B cell.

of immune activation, as it is no longer recognized by T cells. Viruses are often the cause of this type of alteration in cells.

Once activated, T cells will undergo blast transformation and release a large number of soluble mediators. Many of these, grouped as polyclonal B-cell activators, continue the immune response by stimulating B cells, which will form specific antibodies. The antigen may also be destroyed by the action of natural killer cells or macrophages. The immune response can be interrupted at this point by the mechanisms of tolerance.

Tolerance

Tolerance is an effect on activated immune cells that prevents the response to a specific antigen. The response to other antigens remains intact.

It is not clear what role tolerance plays in normal immune function, but it can be viewed as suppressing the immune response to non-self-cells.

The mechanisms of tolerance are shown in outline in Figure 1-5. There are three key elements of the immune response: recognition of the antigen, activation of the immune response and initiating effector mechanisms that destroy the antigen.

Tolerance is usually active at the level of recognition of antigen.

An important example of the role of tolerance is pregnancy. A fetus expresses a blend of MHC that is derived from ovum and sperm. It contains more than enough foreign MHC determinants to trigger immune rejection and destruction of the fetus by maternal immune mechanisms soon after conception. The reasons for this phenomenon are

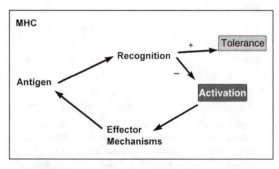

FIGURE 1-5

SUMMARY OF THE OVERALL MECHANISMS FOR DISTINGUISHING ANTIGENS AS SELF AND NON-SELF.

not clear. A form of tolerance is one explanation for maternal immunity ignoring a large foreign graft for the entire duration of pregnancy. One recognized mechanism is that the placenta does not express MHC Class I antigens on the syncytiotrophoblast (closest to maternal circulation) surface. There are alterations in maternal immune function, with down regulation of some immune responses. Pregnancy hormones along with peptides and glycolipids from the placenta also alter immune function.

There are curious paradoxes regarding immune tolerance of the fetus. Women who have had multiple pregnancies, especially with different partners, have very high levels of antibodies to various MHC patterns. Rats that are MHC identical will abort if mated, and the placenta remains small. The more the MHC difference between the rats, the larger the placenta and the better the survival of the fetuses. If maternal cells are placed in culture with irradiated fetal cells, a technique known as a mixed leukocyte reaction, the maternal cells will respond strongly. Finding the answers to this puzzle can help with the understanding of organ transplantation. There may

also be answers that will help in understanding the ultimate failure of immune recognition, cancer.

Recognizing Self

MHC regulation of immune recognition. If MHC Class I antigens match the macrophage MHC library record (upper left) no reaction occurs. If it does not (lower right) the macrophages activate (Figure 1-2).

Immune Surveillance

Among the essential functions of T cells, macrophages, and circulating monocytes is the constant survey of the body for MHC patterns that are deemed foreign. The mechanisms of immune recognition are synthesized into a unified mechanism that surveys the body for foreign antigens and cells that deviate from the MHC that is recognized as self.

This function is diagramed in Figure 1-6. Once activated by a foreign antigen, the immune response cascade is very difficult to stop.

Three main mechanisms are responsible for this survey: MHC recognition, clonal deletion, and anti-idiotypic network (Figure 1-6).

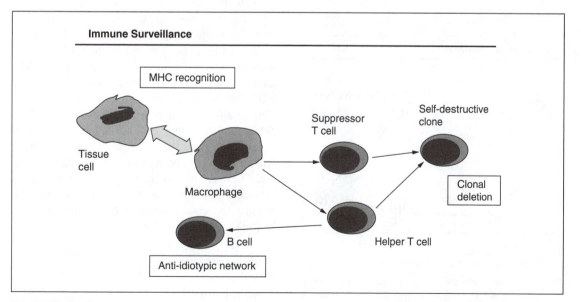

FIGURE 1-6

KEY MECHANISMS IN THE INDUCTION OF TOLERANCE: ALTERED RECOGNITION, ANTI-IDIOTYPE ANTIBODIES, AND CLONAL DELETION.

MHC recognition. The MHC Class I molecules on the surface of all cells are recognized by T cells and macrophages. The T-cell receptor and the MHC Class II structures on the T-cell surface interact with Class I molecules in a highly specific way that is peculiar to each individual.

Clonal deletion. The removal of all cells that display autoreactivity (self-destruction—apoptosis) is the basic function of the thymus. The thymus exerts its maximal effect during embryogenesis, and during this time, 95% of all cells entering the thymus are destroyed because they display autoreactivity or fail to recognize MHC Class I antigens. Following birth, autoregulation is probably by a T-cell network rather than in the thymus.

Anti-idiotypic network. This mechanism of regulation of the immune response was described by Jerne. The anti-idiotypic network is essentially a complex switch that regulates the activity of B cells. In the production of an antibody, normally hidden genetic material is incorporated into the heavy and light chains of the immunoglobulin molecule. The presence of these antigens in circulation results in the production of a second antibody specific for this genetic material. This immune complex forms on the B-cell surface and damps the activity of the cell. A second and third level of anti-antibody will also be formed, leading to a network of antibodies that fine tune the activity of the B cells (Figure 1-7).

T-cell suppressive function. T cells can exert a damping function on the immune response. This activity is important in regulating the reactivity of cells to self-antigens. T cells are capable of down-regulating the function of all immune cells, and in this instance, they block the production of antibodies by B cells and plasma cells.

POLYMORPHONUCLEAR CELLS (PMN)

These cells are derived from the yolk sac of the embryo as early as 3–4 weeks. They function predominantly as scavenger cells. They are drawn toward the site of an immune response by many proteins termed chemoattractants. They ingest antigens that have been *opsonized*. One opsonizing process involves coating the antigen with a protein. This neutralizes the negative charge found on the antigen, preventing the antigen and PMN from repelling each other because of carrying the same electrical charge. Another relies on the binding of antibodies to an antigen so that the portion of the antibody that binds to cells (Fc) is exposed. The antibody thus forms a bridge between the two.

Inflammation occurs mainly because of PMN. This group includes neutrophils and eosinophils. When activated, they produce a large number of inflammatory mediators such as prostaglandins, leukotrienes, IL1, lysozymes, and hydrogen peroxide. These substances are very toxic to organisms that are ingested, but can injure host tissues as well, causing the characteristic signs of inflammation: heat, redness, and swelling.

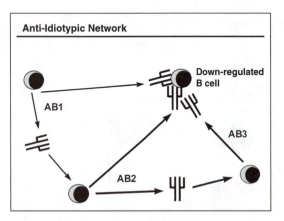

Anti-Idiotypic Network

Down-regulated B cell

AB1

AB2

AB3

FIGURE 1-7

AN ANTI-IDIOTYPIC NETWORK.

The anti-idiotypic network forms in response to the presence of latent antigens on immunoglobulin. These antigens stimulate the formation of an anti-antibody immunoglobulin, which in turn stimulates the formation of a third antibody. This network is thought to regulate B-cell function.

SERUM PROTEINS

Complement

Complement consists of a series of enzymes that derive from each other in a cascade in which each is activated by the previous product. In the process, several smaller, highly potent peptides are produced. These have many actions, such as chemoattraction (Figure 1-8).

There are nine components of the complement pathway, which activate in the sequence: C1,C2,C4,C3,C5,C6,C7,C8,C9. C3 can also be activated by Properdin, also known as the alternate pathway. A general overview of this cascade is shown in Figure 1-8.

The process is initiated by immune complexes which activate C1. The bar lines in the figure indicate activated components. The byproducts C4a, C3a, and C5a are potent chemoattractant molecules, and can be involved in the development of severe shock in a clinical setting. There is an alternate pathway, which bypasses the C1 activation step, and can be activated directly by bacteria.

Complement is a major opsonin, but can also destroy cells directly by damaging the membrane.

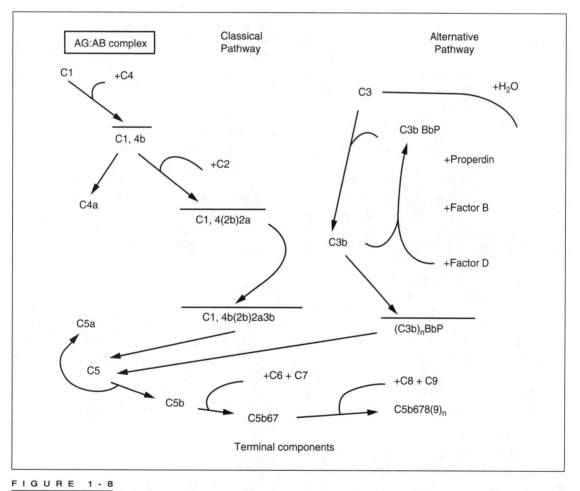

FIGURE 1-8

COMPLEMENT ACTIVATION.

This pathway consists of a series of enzymes in which each activated component activates the next. The classical pathway is activated by antigen-antibody complexes. The alternate pathway is activated directly via C3.

The complex $C_{5b678(9)}$ is the attack complex that is involved in damaging the cell wall of many bacteria (Figure 1-8).

Secondary Immune Organs

The secondary immune organs are the lymph nodes, bone marrow, and the spleen. They are termed secondary, because they are seeded during embryogenesis by newly developed T cells and B cells. The spleen and bone marrow particularly have a structure that is important in mature immune function, while the bone marrow is concerned with production of cells.

Spleen

The splenic white pulp is the site of major immune function. The key structure is the germinal center. Germinal centers are nearly spherical accumulations of lymphocytes. They are arranged with a medulla of B cells and a cortex of T cells. This arrangement allows the maximal amplification of an immune signal, as T cells focus on a large number of B cells. In response to an antigenic stimulus, the germinal centers enlarge as the lymphocytes proliferate in response to the antigen. The spleen may enlarge as a result producing a clinically visible sign of splenomegaly. The splenic white pulp has a unique arrangement of T cells. In addition to the germinal centers, they are arranged along the sinusoids. Blood flow through the white pulp is very slow. An antigen is thus forced to pass slowly through the splenic pulp, allowing a prolonged exposure of the antigen to T cells. This exposure is particularly important for weak antigens, such as polysaccharides. The cell wall of pneumococcus and haemophilus are composed mainly of polysaccharides, and are major pathogens in patients who have had a splenectomy or other splenic pathology as occurs in lymphomatous malignancies.

Lymph Nodes

The arrangement of lymphocytes in lymph nodes is also in germinal centers. As with the spleen, stimulation will cause lymphocytes to proliferate with enlargement of the germinal centers. This response is seen clinically as lymphadenopathy in the drainage path of the site of infection.

REGULATION OF INFECTIOUS AGENTS

The components of the immune system integrate in different ways to eliminate various organisms.

Bacteria

The full array of immune functions outlined above is used to regulate most bacteria. The bacterium is presented to T cells by macrophages. These cells undergo division and stimulate B cells to divide under the influence of polyclonal B-cell activators. Specific clones of cells emerge that are influenced by the presence of the antigen to become plasma cells that produce specific antibodies. These opsonize the bacterium, which is ingested and destroyed by neutrophils. During this process, complement is activated, and in some instances, complement components can destroy the organism.

Mycobacteria

There are notable exceptions to the standard pattern of immune response. *Mycobacterium tuberculosis* is the cause of human tuberculosis, which is possibly the single most important cause of chronic infection worldwide. The immune control of *M. tuberculosis* is exclusively by macrophages and T cells. This has practical implications as it makes the development of a vaccine difficult (Figure 1-9).

Viruses

Viral infections are controlled predominantly be T cells and more specifically by natural killer (NK) cells. These cells produce interferon, which is a key soluble mediator in the destruction of viruses. The degree of antibody production is dependent on the length of time that the virus spends in circulation. This process is diagramed in Figure 1-10.

Fungi

Polymorphonuclear cells are the major defense against fungi, especially in preventing them from entering the blood stream. Some fungi, such as *Candida* sp. are very potent stimulators of T-cell

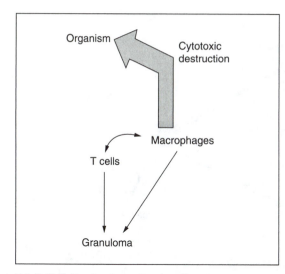

THE IMMUNE CONTROL OF *M. TUBERCULOSIS*.

The immune control of *M. tuberculosis* is exclusively by macrophages and T cells. The macrophages destroy the organism directly, and T cells influence the immune response. Immunoglobulin is not involved. A granuloma, which consists of a central T cell surrounded by epithelialized macrophages, results from this infection.

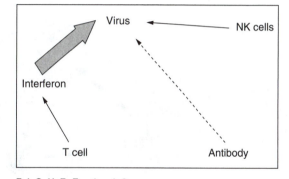

THE ELIMINATION OF VIRUSES.

The elimination of viruses depends on the integrity of the T cell-macrophage axis. Viruses are killed by interferons produced by T cells and macrophages. A very potent subgroup of lymphocytes, natural killer cells (NK cells) is important in destroying cells that are infected by the virus. Antibodies are only produced if the virus spends time in circulation in blood before settling in cells.

responses, but the clearance of these organisms requires antibodies and polymorphonuclear cells. The presence of persistent Candida infection can indicate that T cells are not functional.

Protozoa

These small unicellular organisms do not usually cause infections in humans. When they do, they are regarded as opportunistic and indicate that T cell are not functioning normally. The regulation of these agents is by T cells and macrophages.

Parasites

Large parasites, such as Schistosoma hematobium (a cause of serious and debilitating illness in developing countries), are regulated by IgE. This is the only known beneficial effect of this antibody.

DEVELOPMENT OF THE IMMUNE SYSTEM

Defects in immune function are better understood with a brief exploration of the normal development of the immune system. The essential development process is that of lymphocytes, as this is where the key to the immune response lies. T cells in particular, orchestrate the immune response and control almost all aspects.

All lymphocytes arise from a totipotent stem cell that first gives rise to the lymphoblast series. From this point there is marked divergence in the differentiation into T cells and B cells, which occurs by very different pathways.

T-Cell Development

T cell development is completely dependent on the presence of a functional thymus gland. The precursor lymphoblasts migrate into the developing thymus, where cells that demonstrate autoreactivity are destroyed. The surviving cells reenter circulation and seed the secondary immune organs. See Figure 1-11.

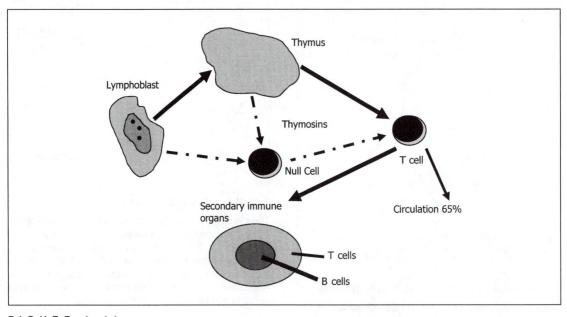

FIGURE 1-11

T-CELL DEVELOPMENT.

In developing into a T cell, the lymphoblast traverses the developing thymus gland. The thymic stroma and T cells develop in tandem. The main function of the thymus during embryogenesis is to educate the T cells to recognize self-antigens.

Thymus

The thymus gland is found in the anterior mediastinum and is in close proximity to the parathyroid glands. The thymus occupies an interesting and incompletely understood place in the emergence of T-cell immunity. It is essential for normal immune development during embryogenesis, but after birth it can be removed without affecting immune function in any obvious way.

Origins

The thymus is derived from the third and fourth branchial pouch of the embryo. It shares this origin with the arch of the aorta and the parathyroid glands.

It consists of stroma and epithelial portions. Areas of the stroma are organized into endocrine tissue called Hassall's corpuscles, where thymosins are formed. These thymosins are a group of substances that convert uncommitted null lymphocytes into T cells at a site distant from the thymus. The best described is factor thymique, but several other forms exist.

After the lymphocytes enter the developing thymus, they progress from the cortex to the medulla in concert with maturation of the thymus. Only 5% of the cells that enter the thymus survive. The main purpose of the passage through the thymus is to ensure that T cells recognize self-MHC and are not activated by it. Any cells that demonstrate auto reactivity undergo apoptosis (programmed self-destruction) and are removed. This development is shown in Figure 1-12.

The course of this progression is from the subcapsular epithelium where the primitive T cells interact with the CTES II thymic epithelial marker. The lymphocytes express the primitive CD1, CD2, and CD5 markers and are CD3, CD4, and CD8 negative. As the cells move into the developing cortex, they encounter CTES III+ epithelium which leads to the development of two populations: CD3−4−8+/CD1−2+5+ and CD3−4+8−/CD1−2+5+. With progression into the medulla and contact with CTES II+IV+, an intermediate population of CD3±4+8− emerges, followed by CD3+4+8+. Finally, with exposure to CTES II+IV+V+ mature T cells are formed with two-thirds being CD3+4+8− and one-third CD3+4−8+.

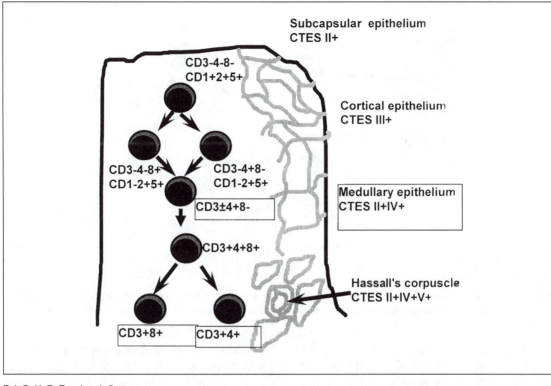

FIGURE 1-12

PASSAGE OF LYMPHOBLASTS THROUGH THE THYMUS.

These cells mature in concert with the stroma of the thymus gland. Over 90% of cells entering the thymus are destroyed because they demonstrate reactivity to self-MHC. The sequence of markers on the T cell and stroma is described in the text.

The mature T cells then migrate to the secondary immune organs and into circulation, where they constitute 60% of lymphocytes. In the secondary immune organs, they constitute the cortex of the germinal centers.

Thymosins from the Hassall's corpuscles (Figure 1-12) act on null cells, causing them to mature into T cells that probably have different characteristics from the cells that become T cells through the thymus.

B-Cell Development

Origin

The emergence of B cells is very different from the development of T cells, and there is far less cell destruction. The emerging lymphoblasts migrate through either the Peyer's patches in the small bowel or the bone marrow. These sites are thought to be analogous to the bursa of Fabricius. Described over 400 years ago, this bursa in the chick embryo is the site of B-cell development (Figure 1-13). During development, the emerging B cells express a range of surface markers, much like T cells. This process is summarized in Figure 1-14. Primitive B cells display CD19, CD9, and CD10. CD9 and CD10 are early markers that are lost, while CD19 persists and is found on mature B cells. A strikingly distinguishing characteristic of developing B cells is the appearance of immunoglobulin. The first to appear is intracytoplasmic IgG, which persists into maturity of the B-cell line.

The focus shifts as the cell matures, and immunoglobulin is found on the cell surface. In an

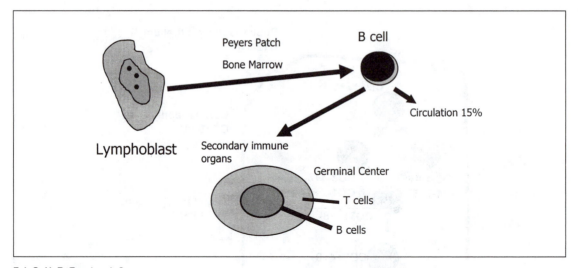

FIGURE 1-13

DEVELOPMENT OF B CELLS.

The process whereby passage through the Peyer's patches and the bone marrow guides lymphoblasts toward becoming B cells is not clear. Mature B cells emerge from the bone marrow and seed the secondary immune organs.

intermediate B cell, there is predominantly IgM with a small amount of IgD on the cell surface. At this stage, cells first express CD5, which seem to have a role in tolerance. As maturation progresses, the surface pattern changes to predominantly IgD, with a small amount of IgM present. Many other structures emerge with specific functions: receptors for complement components, receptors for Fc

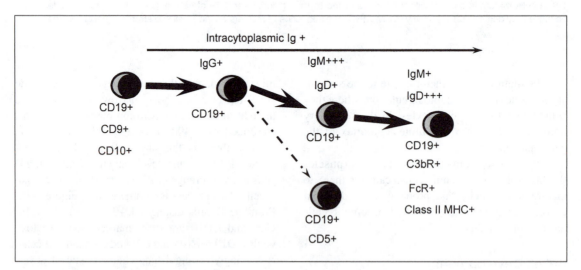

FIGURE 1-14

MARKERS OF MATURATION OF B CELLS.

As B cells mature they express an emerging pattern of surface receptors. The function of these receptors differs from T cells in that many are very specific, for example, the C3b receptor, for complement components.

portions of immunoglobulins, molecules that are the reciprocal for binding to adhesion molecules and Class II MHC (Figures 1-13 and 1-14).

The mature B cell distribute to the medulla of the germinal centers of the secondary immune organs, and constitute 15% of circulating lymphocytes. Unlike T cells, the functional B cells are those in the secondary immune organs. Circulating B cells do not readily produce immunoglobulin in vitro, and do not transform into plasma cells.

Formation of Antibody Producing Cells

B cells undergo a complex further development process to produce antibody forming plasma cells and memory cells that will react to a specific antigen. There are two phases to this process, *clonal development* and *clonal expansion*.

Clonal development. In the secondary immune organs, B cells undergo a unique development, transforming into clones committed to a single antibody isotype. These cells develop first into clones of cells that produce IgM, followed by cells that are IgG clones, and finally clones that produce IgA. During this phase there is rearrangement of the genes on chromosomes 2, 14, and 22. Regions of the light and heavy chain hypervariable regions combine by rearranging the V, D, and J regions into a library of hypervariable region specificities. Immunoglobulins appear in the same order during phylogeny (development of the species or Evolution). With each immune response, immunoglobulins appear in the same sequence, IgM, IgG then IgA. The development of B cells is an example of a situation where ontogeny (development of the individual) repeats phylogeny. This is shown on the left of Figure 1-15.

These clones of cells appear by 10 weeks, when the fetus can make IgM. Clones that produce IgG are present by the middle of the second trimester but the fetus has the ability to make IgA only at term (Table 1-4).

Clonal expansion. After birth, the newborn infant is exposed to a large number of antigens, which initiate an immune response. The clones of B cells that emerged during development are now

TABLE 1-4

SEQUENCE OF APPEARANCE OF CLONES OF B CELLS IN THE FETUS AS WEEKS OF GESTATION

Isotype (cells)	Appearance (weeks)
IgM	10
IgG	30
IgA	40

stimulated and divide rapidly. The first to respond for each antigen are IgM producing cells, then IgG, and then IgA. The IgM response is short-lived, while IgG antibody levels are sustained.

For each of the B-cell responses, there are two populations of daughter cells produced. The first transforms into plasma cells that sort through a gene library to develop a precise fit to the antigen to the hypervariable region of the antibody. The second group becomes memory cells that retain IgD on the surface. This antibody is the switch immunoglobulin that activates these cells when the antigen is encountered again. In this way, an enormous repository of cells is developed that can respond to a wide variety of antigens.

Passive Immunity

Transplacental

Immunoglobulin is present at birth in the newborn. This is passive immunity acquired from the mother. Figure 1-16 shows the transfer of immunoglobulin and the emergence of immunoglobulin in the newborn. Only IgG is transferred across the placenta into the fetus by an active glucose dependent transport mechanism starting at 32 weeks of gestational age. IgM and IgA do not cross the placenta. From birth, the newborn starts to make immunoglobulin in response to antigens, with a gradual increase in IgG, IgM, and IgA. In the meanwhile, maternal IgG decays with a half-life of 30 days, and by 6 months is mostly gone. There is a trough in the level of immunoglobulin at 2–4 months when maternal immunoglobulin is lower, and the newborn infant

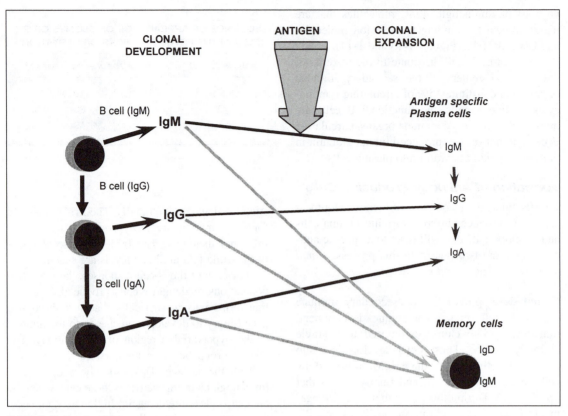

FIGURE 1-15

CONCEPT OF CLONAL DEVELOPMENT AND CLONAL EXPANSION.

Specific clones of B cells emerge, for each isotype. After antigen exposure, the clones expand. This concept is described in the text.

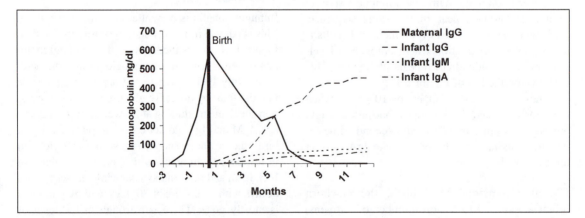

FIGURE 1-16

IMMUNOGLOBULIN LEVELS IN FETAL/NEWBORN PLASMA.

has not yet made adequate levels of antibody. By 1 year, infant immunoglobulin levels are at 60% of adult values (Figure 1-16).

Breast Milk

There are solid data on the protective effects of breast feeding on preventing early infections in infants, especially infantile diarrhea. Severe gastrointestinal infections are a major cause of infant mortality in developing countries, and breast feeding almost completely eliminates this problem. There is transfer of IgA and IgG to the newborn from the first feed. The highest levels of IgA are found in colostrum, where they are 40 times serum levels. The concentration of IgA falls rapidly over the next few days to reach serum levels. The first feeds with colostrum are important for providing specific, protective IgA to the infant.

Early breast milk and colostrum also contains cells. Macrophages and T cell are present. Data from mice indicate that these cells can be found in Peyer's patches, where they may provide antigenic information.

Hemopoietic Cells

The neutrophils, eosinophils, macrophages, and basophils are derived from a totipotent hemopoietic stem cell that in turn derives from the yolk sac early in embryogenesis. The development of these cells is dependent on interleukins and colony forming factors. The specifics of interaction of these molecules are shown in Figure 1-17.

The colony stimulating factors produce colony forming units (CFU) that become increasingly specialized, starting with the totipotent colony, granulocyte-eosinophil-monocyte-macrophage CFU. This evolves into an eosinophil CFU and a granulocyte-monocyte CFU (CFU-GM). CFU-GM gives rise to neutrophils under the influence of IL3, and G-CSF and GM-CSF. The influence of IL3, GM-CSF, and M-CSF produces monocytes, which evolve into the sessile form, macrophages under

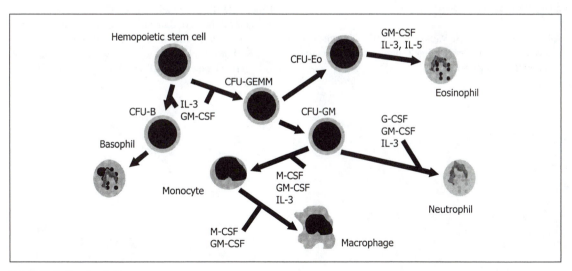

FIGURE 1 - 1 7

FORMATION OF HEMOPOIETIC CELL LINE.

The polymorphonuclear cells emerge from primitive colony forming units. Maturation progresses along the arrows under the influence of colony stimulating factors and interleukins. CFU-B: colony forming unit-basophil; GM-CSF: granulocyte-monocyte colony stimulating factor; M-CSF: monocyte colony stimulating factor; G-CSF: granulocyte colony stimulating factor; CFU-GEMM: colony forming unit-granulocyte-eosinophil-monocyte-macrophage; CFU-GM: colony forming unit-granulocyte-monocyte; IL: interleukin.

further influence of M-CSF in the presence of GM-CSF. The eosinophil CFU is acted on by IL3, IL5, and GM-CSF to develop into mature eosinophils.

Basophils develop directly from the stem cell in response to IL3 and GM-CSF, which produces CFU-B (basophil colony forming units). These evolve directly into basophils, which become the sessile form of the cell, mast cells (Figure 1-17).

CONCLUSION

Immune function is a complex process, with multiple cells and soluble mediators involved at every step. The main recognition mechanism depends on the major histocompatibility complex, which is the identification molecule of the individual at a molecular level.

The development of this system is equally complex, and errors at numerous steps in the formation of immune function during embryogenesis can lead to serious disease.

Suggested Reading

Athanassakis, I. and S. Vassiliadis (2002). T-regulatory cells: are we re-discovering T suppressors? *Immunol Lett* **84**(3): 179–83.

Cooper, M. D. (2002). Exploring lymphocyte differentiation pathways. *Immunol Rev* **185**: 175–85.

Cupedo, T., G. Kraal, et al. (2002). The role of CD45+CD4+CD3– cells in lymphoid organ development. *Immunol Rev* **189**: 41–50.

Defrance, T., M. Casamayor-Palleja, et al. (2002). The life and death of a B cell. *Adv Cancer Res* **86**: 195–225.

Fabbri, M., C. Smart, et al. (2003). T lymphocytes. *Int J Biochem Cell Biol* **35**(7): 1004–8.

Hardy, R. R. (2003). B-cell commitment: deciding on the players. *Curr Opin Immunol* **15**(2): 158–65.

Jones, E., M. Dahm-Vicker, et al. (2003). CD25+ regulatory T cells and tumor immunity. *Immunol Lett* **85**(2): 141–3.

Love, P. E. and A. C. Chan (2003). Regulation of thymocyte development: only the meek survive. *Curr Opin Immunol* **15**(2): 199–203.

Moll, H. (2003). Dendritic cells and host resistance to infection. *Cell Microbiol* **5**(8): 493–500.

Rajnavolgyi, E. and A. Lanyi (2003). Role of CD4+ T lymphocytes in antitumor immunity. *Adv Cancer Res* **87**: 195–249.

Szekeres-Bartho, J. (2002). Immunological relationship between the mother and the fetus. *Int Rev Immunol* **21**(6): 471–95.

Umetsu, D. T., O. Akbari, et al. (2003). Regulatory T cells control the development of allergic disease and asthma. *J Allergy Clin Immunol* **112**(3): 480–7; quiz 488.

von Boehmer, H., I. Aifantis, et al. (2003). Thymic selection revisited: how essential is it? *Immunol Rev* **191**: 62–78.

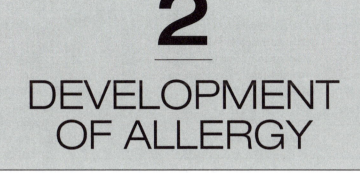

2

DEVELOPMENT OF ALLERGY

ALLERGIC REACTIONS

The pathophysiology of allergic injury is both more complicated and broader in its reach than might appear at first. There are four distinct immunologic mechanisms that give rise to immune injury. They are discussed in this chapter, with clinical examples of each.

The Basis of Allergic Injury

One grouping of allergic reactions was proposed in 1963 by Gell and Coombs. This classification neatly groups allergic (immune) injury into four types according to their pathophysiology. While this is an older classification, it is still useful in categorizing the allergic/immune mechanism behind clinical responses that seem very different from each other but actually share immune activation as the basic mechanism (Table 2-1).

Tyipe I responses are typical of IgE mediated allergic reactions. Types II and III are mediated by IgG directed against a normal cell component (Type II) or against a soluble antigen as immune complexes (Type III). Type IV is completely different, and is regulated by the interaction of macrophages and T cells.

Genetics of Allergic Responses

There is a strong genetic predisposition for allergic responses.

Comparisons of monozygous and dizygous twins shows very high concordance in identical twins (82%) for IgE levels, which is less in dizygous twins (46%). One reason for this discrepancy is that there remains a high influence from the environment. The risk that relatives might develop asthma has been more difficult to calculate, because there are many factors involved, including shared environmental circumstances.

Linked Chromosomes

Several chromosomes have shown strong linkage to IgE levels or to cytokine production.

- Chromosome 5q associations
  - Regulation of IgE
  - Interleukins 3, 4, 5, 9, and 13
  - $Beta_2$-adrenergic receptor
  - Asthma and bronchial hyperreactivity
- Chromosome 6 associations
  - The human major histocompatibility region
  - Eosinophil count

TABLE 2-1

CLASSIFICATION OF THE MECHANISMS OF ALLERGIC INJURY AND EXAMPLES OF EACH ARE PRESENTED IN THIS TABLE

Type	Mechanism	Examples
Type I	IgE mediated allergy	Allergic rhinitis
	Within 30 minutes	Urticaria
Type II	IgG directed against formed cell components	Incompatible blood transfusion
Type III	IgG Immune complex	Serum sickness
		Vasculitis
Type IV	Cell mediated	TB granuloma
	T cell-macrophage	Sarcoidosis

- Chromosome 11q associations
  - High affinity IgE Fc receptor (FcεRIbeta)
- Chromosome 12q associations
  - Afro-Caribbean population
  - Asthma
  - Total IgE levels
  - Amish population
  - Total IgE levels
- Chromosome 13 associations
  - Total serum IgE levels
- Chromosome 14q associations
  - T-cell antigen receptor

TYPE I

Production of IgE

IgE is produced by B cells that transform into plasma cells secreting specific IgE. The basic mechanism is similar to production of antibody in response to an antigen stimulus (Chap. 1, Immune function). The mechanisms that produce a class switch to IgE instead of IgG, IgM, or IgA are only partly understood. One explanation is the interaction of environment and genetics as described in the Hygiene Hypothesis (discussed in Chap. 3)

Several interleukins (IL) influence the B-cell response. The most important of these appears to be IL4, especially in the presence of Th2 type helper cells. Under the combined influence of genetic and cytokine factors, B cells produce IgE that is highly specific for the antigen. Unlike other serum immunoglobulins, IgE functions only when attached to mast cells or basophils. It binds by the Fc portion of the molecule to the high affinity IgE Fc receptor (FcεRI). There is a high density of these receptors on basophils and mast cells. This form of binding leaves the Fab portion free in blood or extracellular fluid where it binds strongly with the antigen when the body next encounters it. The reaction is quite unlike an IgG-antigen reaction, which forms an immune complex in serum.

With the next encounter, the antigen binds to IgE on mast cells, cross-linking two or more IgEs. This action causes perturbation of the membrane, activating membrane enzymes, including phosphorylcholine and phospholipase. This results in opening of calcium channels with an influx of calcium.

Mechanism of Type I

Mast Cells

Mast cells are distinguished by the presence of granules in the cytoplasm. These granules consist of a structural matrix, that contains preformed histamine and eosinophil and neutrophil chemotactic factors (NCF). *NCF* is a component of these granules and is released at the same time as *eosinophil chemotactic factor of anaphylaxis (ECF-A)* and histamine. The disintegration of the granules is controlled by the rate of calcium influx. A small pinocytic vacuole is formed at the membrane which traps a small volume of extracellular fluid. The vacuole migrates to the granules, and dissolves histamine and NCF. It then

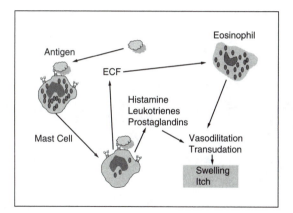

FIGURE 2-1

NORMAL MECHANISM OF THE ALLERGIC RESPONSE.

An antigen attaches to specific IgE that is bound to mast cells. This triggers the release of mediators that cause vasodilatation and transudation of fluid with itching. Further details are explained in the text. ECF: eosinophil chemotactic factors.

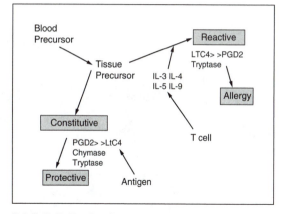

FIGURE 2-2

EMERGENCE OF TWO POPULATIONS OF MAST CELLS FROM BLOOD AND TISSUE PRECURSORS.

The superficial mast cells are reactive and take part in IgE mediated reactions. The deep, constitutive mast cells are part of the normal IgG response.

migrates to the membrane and releases the contents. The severity of the allergic reaction is in proportion to the rapidity of the release of histamine and other mediators (Figure 2-1).

It has recently been noted that there are two types of mast cells: reactive and constitutive. The general function of these mast cells is shown in Figure 2-2.

Reactive mast cells. These cells are found superficially in tissues. They follow the classical path of reaction to antigens noted above. They are under the influence of T cells and especially interleukins 3, 4, 5, and 9, all TH2 type interleukins. In response to antigen binding to IgE, they release histamine and leukotrienes in higher concentration than prostaglandins.

Constitutive mast cells. This type of mast cell is found deep in tissues and has a different range of reactions from the superficial type. In response to an antigen, the cell augments the immune response and releases prostaglandins rather than leukotrienes. They do not take part in the allergic reaction (Figure 2-2).

Other mediators that are released include leukotrienes and prostaglandins, platelet activating factor (PAF), bradykinin, and TNF-α. Together,

prostaglandins and leukotrienes were previously known as the slow reacting substance of anaphylaxis. Both are derived from arachidonic acid, which is catabolized by the action of either cyclooxygenase to prostaglandins or lipoxygenase to leukotrienes. An outline of the pathway is shown in Figure 2-3. The leukotrienes (LT) cascade into LTC4, LTD4, and LTE4. They have major effects, especially in causing increased secretion, increased mucus production, increased interstitial fluid and are chemoattractant for eosinophils. Prostaglandins have similar effects. PGF2α is a bronchodilator, unlike PGE. Thromboxane is an early product of cyclooxygenase activity. It is chemotactic for polymorphonuclear cells and eosinophils (Figure 2-3).

PAF has a direct effect on platelets, stimulating the release of serotonin, which is potently vasoactive.

Eosinophils

These are potent cells that release a number of mediators. They can be very destructive to tissues. In terms of immunologic function, eosinophils are a key defense against parasites such as ascaris or schistosomiasis.

Eosinophils contain two main types of secretory granules: the specific and the small granules. The specific granules contain major basic protein

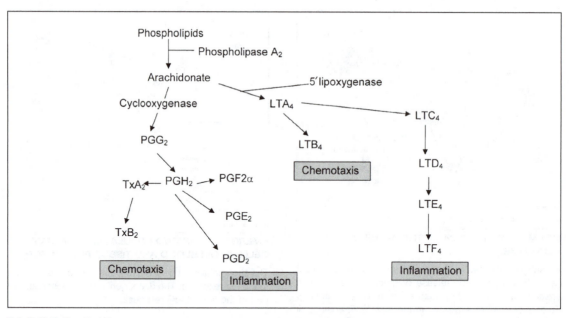

FIGURE 2-3

SCHEMA OF PRODUCTION OF LEUKOTRIENES AND PROSTAGLANDINS.

PG: prostaglandin; Tx: thromboxane; LT: leukotriene. In general, the early products of arachidonic acid catabolism are chemotactic (TxB2 and LTB4), while later components produce inflammation.

(MBP) (55% of the granule), eosinophil cationic protein (ECP), eosinophil-derived neurotoxin (EDN), and beta-glucuronidase. The small granules contain enzymes, including acid phosphatase and arylsulfatase B.

Eosinophil chemotaxis. Eosinophils accumulate rapidly at the site of an allergic response. This is due to a number of mediators, including ECF-A and NCF and histamine.

Effects of the Mediators

Histamine. Histamine is a vasodilator and causes transudation of fluid into the extracellular space. If it is released rapidly enough, as would occur in an anaphylactic reaction, there will be marked and rapid vasodilatation, leading to hypovolemic shock. This can occur in patients who are allergic to peanuts, for example. Histamine will also cause constriction of smooth muscle of the airways, leading to potentially severe bronchospasm. Transudation of fluid into the extracellular space will lead to *edema*, and, in the skin, to urticaria and angioedema. Because the fluid accumulates in the superficial layers of skin or mucosa, there is stimulation of the fine nerve endings, leading to *itch*. In the nose, the release of histamine will also cause rhinorrhea, sneezing and, to a lesser extent, nasal blockage.

Beta-chemokines

Histamine releasing factors. Histamine releasing factors (HRFs) may also be responsible for the protracted non-IgE-dependent histamine release seen in late phase reactions. They are products of neutrophils, platelets, alveolar macrophages, and T cells and B cells. The various forms of HRF have now been identified to correspond to the members of the beta-chemokine group of cytokines. HRF activates target cells.

Other chemokines

- Monocyte chemotactic and activating factor (MCAF)/monocyte chemotactic peptide-1 regulated on activation, normal T-cell expressed and secreted (RANTES)
- Macrophage inflammatory peptides
- Eotaxin

Biphasic Reaction

Early

The immediate allergic reaction occurs within 30 minutes of exposure, but often occurs in minutes. Usually, the more rapidly the onset occurs, the more severe the clinical reaction. This reaction is mediated by:

- Histamine
- Kinins
- Leukotrienes
- Superoxide free radicals
- Prostaglandins

These mediators have in common that they have effects on the vasculature, causing vasodilatation and edema, bronchospasm and increased mucus secretion.

Late

The late reaction involves cells, particularly eosinophils and neutrophils. This reaction is mediated by the following:

- Eosinophils
- Neutrophils
- Basophils
- Monocytes
- T-lymphocytes

Mediators that are involved are similar to the acute phase and include the following:

- Histamine
- Kinins
- Leukotrienes
- Superoxide free radicals

In the late phase, the leukotrienes are much more active than histamine. Prostaglandins seem not to play a part in the late phase reaction.

The early and late reactions are presented schematically in Figure 2-4.

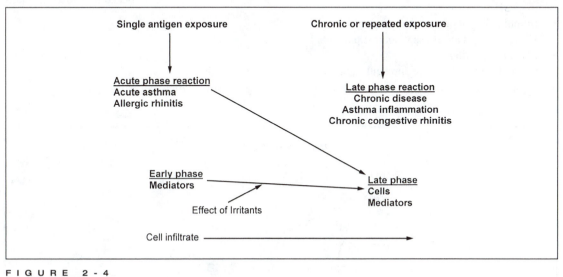

F I G U R E   2 - 4

SCHEMA OF THE EARLY AND LATE ALLERGIC REACTIONS.

This response is on a continuum. A single exposure of the antigen leads to an immediate response that is mediated by histamine and other vasoactive substances. Repeated exposure to an antigen results in an eosinophilic infiltrate. The late response can also be caused by innate properties of the antigen.

TYPE II

This is a common form of allergic injury with diverse presentations.

Mechanism

This is an IgG mediated reaction. Compared to the Type I reaction, it is straightforward. There is an immune reaction against a normal cell component.

Examples

- Blood group incompatibilities
  - IgG is directed against the ABO blood group. This results in destruction of incompatible blood cells
- Goodpasture's syndrome
  - IgG directed against basement membrane gives rise to renal and pulmonary disease
- Pemphigus
  - IgG is directed against various skin components, giving rise to bullous lesions
- Bullous pemphigoid
- Graves' disease
  - Antibody functions in a similar manner to TSH
- Immune thrombocytopenic purpura
  - Antibodies are present against platelets
- Myasthenia gravis
  - IgG antibodies are present against the acetylcholine receptor

TYPE IIA

Clinical Presentation

An eight-year-old male presents with a macular erythematous facial rash.

He had been on a hiking outing with his family. He has been using sunscreen. The rash is distributed over his face and neck in the V of his shirt. He has similar lesions on his legs that stop at the line of his short pants. His reaction is a photosensitive dermatitis, in which there is an IgG reaction against collagen that has been altered by the combined action of sunlight and the presence of para amino benzoic acid.

Mechanism

This reaction is a modification of Type II in which there is an immune response against an altered cell surface.

This reaction is based on immune complex formation with resultant vasculitis. An antigen stimulates IgE production with histamine release; this mediator opens the endothelial junctions. Antigen remains in excess and produces soluble complexes with IgG which deposit in the subendothelial space. Complement is activated and vascular damage ensues (Figure 2-5).

Examples

- Hepatitis
  - Target: MHC on hepatocyte

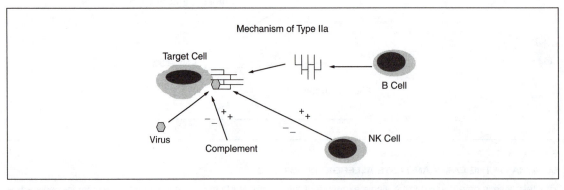

FIGURE 2-5

TYPE IIA REACTION.

MHC on the cell surface is altered by a virus. Macrophages are activated and initiate a destructive immunological response.

- Photosensitive dermatitis
  - Target: skin collagen

TYPE III

This is an immune complex reaction that is IgG mediated. Immune complexes form in the presence of antigen excess, and remain soluble instead of forming an insoluble lattice. These soluble complexes are large and do not cause damage at this stage. In the next phase, there is production of IgE and release of histamine. The histamine increases the gap between endothelial cells, allowing the large complexes to deposit in the subendothelial space. Complement is activated, releasing C3a and C5a. These complement components attract polymorphonuclear cells to the subendothelial space in blood vessels. This influx results in vasculitis (Figure 2-6).

Examples

Hypersensitivity Pneumonitis

In this condition, there is a pulmonary reaction to an inhalant antigen. The response is IgG mediated and results in an immune complex response in the vascular and perivascular space of the lungs. Antigens that give rise to this response include the following:

- Mold spores, e.g., thermophylic actinomycetes
- Insects such as grain weevil
- Industrial compounds that include divalent cations
- Wood dusts, especially cedar and redwood
- Pigeon droppings

Clinical Presentation

The onset of symptoms is usually within 4–6 hours of exposure

Acute

- Flu-like illness
- Fever (may be as high as 104°F)
- Cough
- Dyspnea is often a presenting feature
- Flu-like illness
- Infiltrative pulmonary lesions

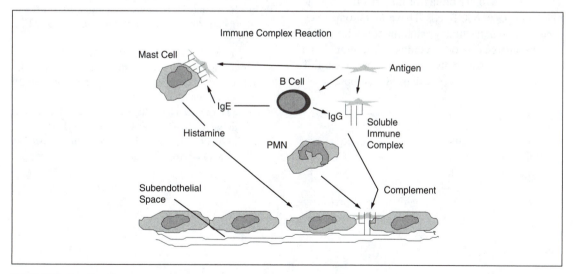

FIGURE 2-6

THE MECHANISM OF TYPE III REACTION.

This reaction is based on immune complex formation with resultant vasculitis. An antigen stimulates IgE production with histamine release; this mediator opens the endothelial junctions. Antigen remains in excess and produces soluble complexes with IgG which deposit in the subendothelial space. Complement is activated and vascular damage ensues.

Chronic

- This form has a much more insidious onset
- Patients may present with progressive dyspnea
- Low-grade fever is often a presenting feature
- Chronic disease may lead to fibrosis
- In the most chronic form, patients are not recognized until the disease has progressed to an end-stage lung disease

Diagnosis

Circulating specific IgG antibodies

- Thermophyllic actinomycetes
- Grain dust
- Pigeon droppings
- Serum sickness

Other causes

- Autoimmune disease
- Celiac disease

TYPE IV

This reaction is the result of the interaction of T cells and macrophages. Antibodies are not involved. There may be direct killing of the organism by the macrophages or NK T cells. These are chronic reactions that often result in granuloma formation, as is seen in tuberculosis or sarcoidosis. The granuloma of sarcoidosis is actually formed from a central T cell with surrounding epithelialized macrophages.

Examples

- Contact dermatitis
- Poison ivy

- Infections
  - Tuberculosis
  - Listeria monocytogenes
- Sarcoidosis

Suggested Reading

Blumenthal MN (2004). New thoughts regarding the genetics of atopy. *Am J Respir Crit Care Med* **169**(5): 555–6.

Bochner, B. S. and R. P. Schleimer (2001). Mast cells, basophils, and eosinophils: distinct but overlapping pathways for recruitment. *Immunol Rev* **179**: 5–15.

Kassel, O. and A. C. Cato (2002). Mast cells as targets for glucocorticoids in the treatment of allergic disorders. *Ernst Schering Res Found Workshop* (40): 153–76.

Pawankar, R. (2001). Mast cells as orchestrators of the allergic reaction: the IgE-IgE receptor mast cell network. *Curr Opin Allergy Clin Immunol* **1**(1): 3–6.

Piliponsky, A. M., G. J. Gleich, et al. (2002). Effects of eosinophils on mast cells: a new pathway for the perpetuation of allergic inflammation. *Mol Immunol* **38**(16–18): 1369.

Robbie-Ryan, M. and M. Brown (2002). The role of mast cells in allergy and autoimmunity. *Curr Opin Immunol* **14**(6): 728–33.

Taylor, M. L. and D. D. Metcalfe (2001). Mast cells in allergy and host defense. *Allergy Asthma Proc* **22**(3): 115–9.

Tokura, Y., M. Rocken, et al. (2001). What are the most promising strategies for the therapeutic immunomodulation of allergic diseases? *Exp Dermatol* **10**(2): 128–37; discussion 138–40.

Venarske D. deShazo RD (2003). Molecular mechanisms of allergic disease. *South Med J* **96**(11): 1049–54.

Yi, E. S. (2002). Hypersensitivity pneumonitis. *Crit Rev Clin Lab Sci* **39**(6): 581–629.

C H A P T E R

3

A NEW PARADIGM: THE HYGIENE HYPOTHESIS

BACKGROUND

An increase has been noted in asthma and allergies in the United States. There are several theories to explain this phenomenon. The current paradigm on the development of asthma as a linear phenomenon does not seem to explain newer data on the emergence of asthma and allergies. These data have suggested a new concept, based on immune maturation that has been termed the hygiene hypothesis. This rethinking of the pathophysiology of asthma has led to a concept of asthma beginning in childhood, irrespective of when symptoms may become manifest.

NEW CONCEPTS OF T-CELL DEVELOPMENT

This concept is shown in Figure 3-1. An uncommitted T helper cell or a Th0 cell matures under the influence of genetic factors, most of which have not been determined. Environmental agents further modulate this maturation. Exposure to bacterial, viral, and other antigens drives this cell to mature into a Th1 cell. These Th1 cells are defined by the production of cytokines that drive B cells to produce defense immunoglobulins: IgG, IgM, and IgA. These key cytokines are interleukin 2 (IL2), tumor necrosis factor, and gamma interferon.

Under other conditions, that have not been fully defined, the drive is for the Th0 cell to mature into a Th2 cell. The presence of antigen and IL4 is one described mechanism that will drive development in this direction. The characteristics of this population of cells are the production of a set of cytokines (IL4, IL5, and IL13) that drive B cells to produce IgE. Currently, there are a limited number of surface markers that differentiate a Th1 from Th2 cell. An essential aspect of the hygiene hypothesis is the concept that newborn infants have a preponderance of Th2 cells. According to this theory, it is exposure to antigens following delivery that drives the development toward Th1. There is a role for genetic input, but the mechanism is not known. Several gene loci have a strong link to the production of IgE, but the mechanism whereby they influence clonal switching is not completely delineated (Figure 3-1).

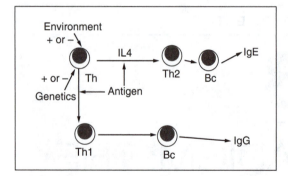

FIGURE 3-1

PROPOSED PATHWAY OF DEVELOPMENT OF T HELPER (Th) CELLS INTO Th1 OR Th2 CELLS.

The development is influenced by genetics and environment as discussed in the text.

APPLICATION OF THE HYGIENE HYPOTHESIS

Asthma and Allergy Development

Figure 3-2 compares the current concept of the genesis of asthma (left arm) with the newer hygiene hypothesis construct (right arm). A central concept

for the new paradigm is a theoretical ideal of immune development in the newborn. This is based on theoretical T-cell populations, which have been identified in mice and inferred from their cytokine profile (Figure 3-2).

The basic pathway of asthma development is identical for both hypotheses and is shown in the center of Figure 3-2. This depends on a genetic predisposition for the disease which is ultimately the reason for development of asthma and allergies. The standard pathophysiology is on the left. This pathway presupposes that there is a genetic predisposition that is acted on by early exposure to allergens and viral infections.

Traditional Pathway

Fitting this concept into the Th1–Th2 hypothesis suggests that early exposure to antigens, such as cockroach and house dust mites, block the transition from Th2 to Th1 cells, allowing the development of IgE and increasing the risk of allergies and asthma. There are well-documented risks of early exposure to cockroaches and dust mites, and some studies have shown risks as high as sixfold for dust mite

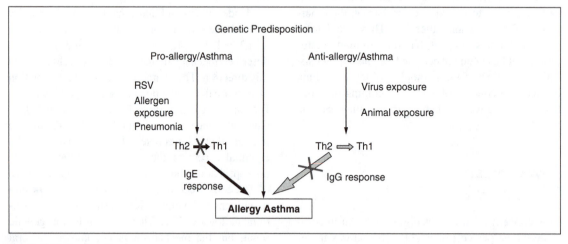

FIGURE 3-2

TRADITIONAL (LEFT ARM) AND HYGIENE (RIGHT ARM) THEORIES OF THE DEVELOPMENT OF ALLERGIES AND ASTHMA.

The central concept of this hypothesis is the transition of Th2 to Th1 T cells. Genetic predisposition underlies the development of atopy. The left hand path depicts the pro atopic effects of infections and allergens. This traditional concept promotes allergy development, possibly by inhibiting Th2 to Th1 development. The right side of the figure shows the anti-allergy aspects of infection and animal exposure, which promote the transition of Th2 to Th1 cells.

exposure. There are data to indicate that early exposure to mold spores and cockroaches are also significant risk factors for the development of asthma.

Another early risk factor is pneumonia. Children who had pneumonia under the age of 3 years have a 3.3 fold risk of developing asthma by 6 years, and 2.8 fold risk by 11 years. Even in the case of lower respiratory tract infection without pneumonia in the same group of children, there was a 2.4 fold risk of asthma at 6 years and 1.6 fold at 11 years. Presumably this infection was due to respiratory syncytial virus (RSV). There is a large body of literature that demonstrates the association of RSV in infancy with the emergence of asthma later in life. Other pulmonary inflammatory viruses can cause similar effects, such as adenovirus or parainfluenza.

There is probably an increased risk for having asthma among patients who have allergies. The genetic alleles that have the strongest link to asthma also have an association with the development of allergies. Studies have shown that the presence of allergic rhinitis is associated with an increased risk of developing asthma that correlates with severity of the rhinitis. There is also an increased risk for children with atopic dermatitis.

Development Along the Hygiene Hypothesis

The development arm that is shown on the right in Figure 3-2 takes an opposing view that represents the hygiene hypothesis. The basis of this theory is that early exposure to antigens such as cat and dog dander and insect antigens increases the transition from Th2 to Th1 type lymphocytes, reducing the emergence of allergies. Early viral and bacterial exposure also increases Th1 cell population, decreasing the risk of the development of allergic diatheses. There is thus a shift toward IgG production, rather than IgE.

COMMENTS ON THE HYGIENE HYPOTHESIS CONTROVERSY

Causes of Allergy Increase

Several new early childhood risk factors for the development of asthma and allergies have now come under consideration.

- Lifestyle
- SES
- Allergen exposure
- Sibship size
- Early childhood infections
- Diet
- Farming environment

CONCEPTS UNDERLYING THE HYGIENE HYPOTHESIS

This hypothesis has pointed out the need for new thinking about the emergence of allergies and asthma. The root of this theory is the balance of Th1 and Th2 cells, but these cells are defined by secondary criteria, i.e., the cytokines that are found in plasma. This makes direct evidence difficult to obtain, and the majority of studies that support this concept are rooted in population statistics rather than immunology. A problem with many of the studies is that they rely on recall data gathered by questionnaire. Conditions that have been linked to a reduction in the development of allergies and asthma are:

- Early exposure to allergens, especially animals
- Early viral infections
- Farm life with barn exposure

Animal Exposure

There is a large body of literature that looks at early animal exposure. For instance, a study from Sweden examined a large number ($n = 2841$) of children and used a questionnaire to determine allergic rhinitis, asthma and allergy test positive. There was a lower frequency of allergic rhinitis at 7 years and of asthma at 12 years. There was a lower incidence of positive allergy test in the animal exposed group. Whether this difference is related to reported animal exposure in the first year of life or other factors is not clear with this study design. In many of the studies that explore this question, there is no independent confirmation of the diagnosis of allergic rhinitis or asthma. The data are collected by recall questionnaires, often completed unaided. The studies are often from Scandinavian countries and Germany, with a more homogenous population, which may imply a different mechanism. Also, genetic factors probably play a major role in the different presentations and are difficult to address.

The data from this group of studies indicate a need for caution in interpretation. There are some recent studies that look at serum cytokines, and show a small increase in Th1 type cells as judged by plasma cytokines.

More data are needed to assess causality or show a relationship between early animal exposure and the prevention of atopy. There does not seem to be enough strong evidence at this time to advise parents to expose young children to animals in the expectation that it will protect against the development of allergies or asthma.

Farm Animals and Endotoxin

There is a body of data that indicate that children who are exposed to barn animals early have a lower incidence of allergies or asthma. These are also mostly recall questionnaire studies, but there are striking associations in some of these studies indicating that farmers' children exposed early to endotoxin and farm animals had reduce frequencies of allergies and asthma. Endotoxin is a lipopolysaccharide that is derived from bacteria, mostly gram negative, and is a potent cause of shock in infections with these organisms. These data again are population based, and show a temporal relationship. They do not necessarily demonstrate causality.

Data from Sweden among a farming community where there are few antibiotics used—children are not routinely vaccinated and have a diet that has a high lactobacillus content—suggest that there is a lower incidence of allergic rhinitis, asthma, and acute hospital visits. One should be cautious in drawing sweeping conclusions from such studies. The data in these studies are self-reported, and the study design does not clearly indicate that the avoidance of antibiotics is the cause. Avoiding vaccinations is potentially dangerous, and stronger data would be needed to take such a step. Diseases that are routinely vaccinated for—measles, mumps,

pertussis, diphtheria, and tetanus—carry a high morbidity and mortality that far outweighs the problems of allergy.

Early Infection

A number of investigators have addressed the issue of early infections and protection against the development of allergies. Many rely on questionnaire information. A school survey suggested that there was a significant increase in the risk of developing asthma if antibiotics were used in the first year, and the risk increased with multiple courses. If the antibiotics were given later, there was no increase in the asthma risk. These data show an association between antibiotic use and asthma; they do not demonstrate a causal relationship. The association with infections and allergies and asthma was strengthened by data from Martinez and coworkers who showed that a higher number of older siblings endowed a protective effect against developing allergies and asthma. The same phenomenon was noted with children entering day care. Those who were younger than 6 months had early wheezing that improved after the age of 5 years, while those who entered day care later developed persistent wheeze. These data support the complex nature of the development of allergies and asthma.

Endotoxin

Endotoxin is a product from the cell wall of bacteria. The major component is lipopolysaccharide, which has demonstrated properties in stimulating T cells and inducing cell proliferation. This is also the bacterial component that is responsible for the development of shock in gram negative sepsis. Data from farming communities indicate that there is an increase in gamma interferon among children exposed early to high levels of dust endotoxin. There are other sets of data that indicate that there is an increase in asthma with exposure to endotoxin laden dust. The implication is that the response of an infant to allergens and immune stimulants depends on a number of factors including genetics and timing of exposure.

Breast Milk Protection

There are studies that suggest a protective effect of breast milk in reducing the frequency of allergies and asthma.

Infants with genetic propensity for allergy have shown reduced expression of allergies when breast fed longer than 3 months, and solid foods were introduced late. There are other similar studies, with modest odds ratios suggesting a protective effect.

One difficulty with performing studies on breast feeding and allergies is that it is very difficult, if not impossible to breast feed exclusively. The reason is that minute quantities of foods in the mother's diet cross into breast milk, exposing the newborn to potentially sensitizing doses of antigens. It is theoretically possible that the infant may become sensitized, rather than being protected by breast milk.

In an attempt to address these problems, the effect of feeding hydrolyzed formula was studied. Cow's milk and eggs were not given during the first year. There seemed to be a lasting effect in reducing allergies that correlated with the degree to which the formula was hydrolyzed, with the maximal effect seen with complete hydrolysis of the formula.

Season of Birth

Does the season in which a child is born affect the risk of developing allergies? A group of Swedish investigators examined this question. Their data from 200 children suggested that being born in the spring in Sweden reduced the risk of allergic rhinoconjunctivitis and a positive screen for specific IgE. On the other hand, being born in the winter increased the risk of having allergies and asthma. While there are many factors that could account for this pattern, it is possible that children born in the winter had greater antigen exposure because of being indoors.

Findings in cord blood

The cord blood of atopic mothers was studied in vitro. When cultured under appropriate conditions, the T cells developed into Th2 like clones of T cells that produced IL4 and IL5. There was no predictive correlation noted for development of these clones. Another group of studies demonstrated that there was no correlation between IL12 production by cord blood mononuclear cells and subsequent atopy. There was increased IL12 production to specific proteins such as cat antigen in these studies but this finding did not have a predictive value.

Investigators have found there are higher cord blood levels of CD4+ cells in children born to atopic mothers. Functional studies suggest that there may be delayed T-cell maturation.

It seems from these studies that there are some predictive patterns in cord blood. More investigation is needed to delineate the early changes in newborn immune response that may predict the subsequent development of allergies. Since neither IgE nor IgA cross the placenta, levels of IgA in cord blood have been used as a marker to exclude contamination of fetal blood by maternal at the time of placental separation. There is some debate regarding the level of IgA that is acceptable. IgE levels in cord blood predicted urticaria to food.

Outcome of wheezing

From a large data set, Martinez and coworkers have determined that there are two groups of children under the age of 6 years who present with wheezing. Roughly half will no longer have problems after the age of 6, while the other half will continue with asthma symptoms and acute episodes. The group that continues to have problems has a family history of asthma and allergies, and demonstrates evidence of atopy by history. These features are also found in children who only start to have wheezing symptoms after the age of 6 years, but then continue with frequent asthma episodes into adulthood.

A very long-term study from Australia followed asthmatics for over 30 years. There were two groups of patients. Those whose symptoms resolved were thought to have had a prolonged pulmonary inflammatory response to viral infections and were akin to the children described by Martinez who improved by age 6 years. Those with asthma seemed to remain true to their initial presentation. Those with a severe initial presentation continued to have severe asthma throughout the course of the study. On the other hand, mild asthmatics remained mild throughout the course of the study. These data argue for a strong genetic influence over environmental factors.

CONSIDERATION OF PREDICTING SEVERE DISEASE

Another practical consideration is the risk of a severe outcome for asthma. There have been several attempts to categorize the patients at risk for a poor outcome. From a clinical perspective, having reliable criteria to anticipate the patient who is likely to have a severe asthmatic episode can improve the management of these patients. There are some predictors that are useful to a clinician.

Distilling several profiles of the risk factors for a poor asthma outcome reveals common situations that place the patient at risk.

Number of Medications

The more medications that are needed for control, the greater the risk of a severe episode.

A patient who is taking >3 groups of asthma medications was shown to have an increase in severe episodes of asthma.

Compliance

Two forms of compliance have been considered. The patient who does not take medication as prescribed is at risk. The other example of poor compliance is the failure to keep scheduled appointments. The clinician should regard these as warning signs of a patient who is at severe risk of morbidity and mortality. The patient's knowledge of medication and self-management options should be assessed at each visit. Patients in this category should be reminded of visits by several means, and social services involved where possible.

Self-Management

In chronic diseases like asthma that can have frequent life-threatening episodes, the more a patient understands the concepts of self-management of the

disease, the better the outcome. In asthma, improved outcome for an acute episode correlates with the speed with which a patient receives a bronchodilator. Teaching patients asthma self-management has been shown to be a simple procedure that produces a significant reduction in severe episodes and hospitalizations.

High Risk Factors

Tobacco Use

Some estimates place tobacco use as responsible for one-third of all preventable diseases. Both primary and secondary cigarette smoking increase the severity of lung disease and aggravate upper airway conditions such as sinusitis. Many studies have shown that smoking is a major risk factor in asthma. Smoking marijuana may actually cause more severe effects, as the smoke is unfiltered and is often held in the lungs far longer.

Chronic Exposure to Antigens

Large population based studies such as the National Cooperative Inner-City Asthma Study, have shown the sharp increase in asthma severity among patients chronically exposed to antigens including mold and cockroaches. Having furry animals also emerges as a risk factor.

CONCLUSIONS

The current status of the hygiene hypothesis is an indicator of the complexity of the development of allergies and asthma. The pathophysiology of these conditions is unlikely to be contained in a single concept. There are currently diametrically opposed data that indicate that early exposure to animal dander can reduce or increase the incidence of asthma and allergies. Both are likely to be correct, and depend on circumstances that have yet to be defined. The current concepts can be considered as high antigen load or low antigen load.

High Antigen Theory

This presupposes that early exposure to potent antigens, such as cat dander, increases the risk of developing allergies and asthma. Under this theory, one would advise a patient to

Avoid animals

Remove antigens

Minimize early viral infections

Early use of medications

Low Antigen Theory

This theory supports the concept that early exposure to allergens moves the immune response away from an allergic Th2 type response toward a Th1 based IgG class switch. By this theory, it is better to

Have more pets when the infant is young

Children should have the opportunity to be exposed to farm animals and endotoxin early in life

No antibiotics

No immunizations

Large families are preferable perhaps because the presence of many children increases the risk of infection

Early airway infections are protective

Suggested Reading

Chan-Yeung, M., L. X. Zhan, et al. (2002). The prevalence of asthma and asthma-like symptoms among adults in rural Beijing, China. *Eur Respir J* **19**(5): 853–8.

Chu, H. W., J. M. Honour, et al. (2003). Effects of respiratory Mycoplasma pneumoniae infection on allergen-induced bronchial hyperresponsiveness and lung inflammation in mice. *Infect Immun* **71**(3): 1520–6.

Flohr, C. (2003). Dirt, worms and atopic dermatitis. *Br J Dermatol* **148**(5): 871–7.

Holla, A. D., S. R. Roy, et al. (2002). Endotoxin, atopy and asthma. *Curr Opin Allergy Clin Immunol* **2**(2): 141–5.

Kemp, A. and B. Bjorksten (2003). Immune deviation and the hygiene hypothesis: a review of the epidemiological evidence. *Pediatr Allergy Immunol* **14**(2): 74–80.

Liu, A. H. and J. R. Murphy (2003). Hygiene hypothesis: fact or fiction? *J Allergy Clin Immunol* **111**(3): 471–8.

Offit, P. A. and C. J. Hackett (2003). Addressing parents' concerns: do vaccines cause allergic or autoimmune diseases? *Pediatrics* **111**(3): 653–9.

Sheikh, A., L. Smeeth, et al. (2003). There is no evidence of an inverse relationship between Th2-mediated atopy and Th1-mediated autoimmune disorders: lack of support for the hygiene hypothesis [comment]. *J Allergy Clin Immunol* **111**(1): 131–5.

von Mutius, E. (2001). Infection: friend or foe in the development of atopy and asthma? The epidemiological evidence [comment]. *Eur Respir J* **18**(5): 872–81.

4

ATOPIC DERMATITIS

GENERAL

There is overlap in the use of the term atopic dermatitis (AD) and eczema and neither condition is clearly defined. It is probably most useful to consider eczema as a form of atopic dermatitis. Both conditions are a response of the skin to irritant stimuli of various types. The result of this stimulation is an inflammatory skin response, that results in drying of the skin and hyperkeratosis. Other features include erythema and vesiculation which occur acutely. AD is defined as an inherited, chronic, recurrent, and pruritic form of eczema. There is often an association with other allergic diseases, such as allergic rhinitis and asthma. The condition is unusual in that the pruritus is the cause of the lesions, not the result. Most of the skin lesions occur from repeated trauma in the form of scratching.

TYPICAL PATHOLOGY OF ATOPIC DERMATITIS

Acute

In acute lesions, there are minimal changes seen, mostly intercellular edema of the epidermis and intracellular edema. A sparse lymphocytic infiltrate can be noted in the epidermis. More marked changes are seen in the dermis, with a perivenular infiltrate consisting of lymphocytes and monocytes. Eosinophils, basophils, and neutrophils are sparse.

Chronic

In chronic AD, there is a more prominent lymphocytic infiltrate into the dermis.

These cells are predominantly CD3, CD4, and CD45RO (memory) T cells. They are activated as measured by expression of CD25 and HLA-DR surface antigens. Infiltrating T cells infiltrating into atopic skin lesions express high levels of the skin cutaneous lymphocyte antigen (CLA), a ligand for the vascular adhesion molecule, E-selectin. The skin in chronic AD displays lichenified lesions with prominent hyperkeratosis. In addition, there are increased numbers of epidermal Langerhans' cells and infiltration by monocytes and macrophages. Mast cells are found in various stages of disintegration. Vascular endothelial cells within the lesions express high levels of the adhesion molecule, E-selectin, as well as vascular cell adhesion molecule-1 (VCAM-1). The migration of these inflammatory cells is probably mediated by high levels of the cytokine mediators, interleukin1 and TNF-α.

PATHOPHYSIOLOGY

An irritative stimulus is the initiating event in atopic dermatitis. This can be exposure to an allergen, a chemical or heavy metal, but almost any stimulus can trigger a response in a sensitive individual. Over 80% of patients with atopic dermatitis have elevated IgE in serum or positive in vivo allergy tests, and there is evidence to suggest an etiologic relationship between serum IgE or positive allergy skin tests and atopic dermatitis.

Immune Alterations

IgE is increased in serum and there is an increase in proallergic cytokines (IL4, IL5, IL10). There is an increase in expression of mRNA for IL4 and IL5, indicating that the genes for these mediators are activated. There is a decrease in cytokines that reduce the production of IgE (IL2, IFN-γ). Delayed hypersensitivity cutaneous response is reduced. This is a response that is mediated by T cells. The peak of the reaction is seen 48–72 hours after application of the antigen to the skin. Eosinophils appear to play a greater role in chronic lesions than in acute and are more prominent in chronic lesions. A key cytotoxic product of eosinophils, major basic protein, is deposited prominently in involved areas compared to uninvolved skin. A second product, eosinophil cationic protein, is elevated in serum of patients with AD and levels correlate with disease severity. There is an imbalance of lymphocyte subtypes, with an infiltrate that is predominantly CD3+4+ (helper type) T cells with sparse CD3+8+ (suppressor type).

The situation is not clearly a reflection of an excess of Th2 (proallergy) cytokines, as patients with chronic lesions had increased numbers of IL12 mRNA-positive cells compared with acute and uninvolved skin. IL12 is a potent inducer of IFN-γ synthesis which is a key cytokine in suppression of IgE production.

Similarities in the allergic inflammation of asthma and AD have been noted. There is local infiltration of Th2-like cells in response to allergens, development of specific IgE to allergens, a chronic inflammatory process, and organ-specific

hyperreactivity. Eosinophil recruitment is central to both processes. In addition, epidermal Langerhans' cells in AD skin express IgE on their cell surface. These cells are significantly more efficient than IgE-negative Langerhans' cells at presenting allergen to T cells. Langerhans' cells from atopic individuals have a much higher expression of IgE receptor.

T-cell effector function in AD is closely linked to the ability to express CLA. Where patients have milk-induced AD, there are significantly higher levels of CLA to casein than to other antigens, demonstrating the role of these cells. Other studies indicate that skin reactions to antigens such as dust mites are mediated by the CLA-expressing fraction of T cells. Moreover, these cells isolated from patients with AD but not from normal controls showed evidence of activation (HLA-DR expression) and also spontaneously produced IL4 but not IFN-γ.

Toxins, such as staphylococcal toxin, can induce CLA expression by stimulating IL12 production. In addition, other staphylococcal proteins such as protein A and alpha toxin can participate in the induction of local inflammation in AD by releasing TNF-α from epidermal keratinocytes. Toxins also stimulate a high number of T cells via the T-cell receptor beta-chain, causing amplification of the T-cell response. Persistent cutaneous inflammation could be a result of amplifying T-cell pathways.

An important factor in the emergence of eczema, is the itch-scratch cycle. Repeated trauma to the keratinocytes results in the release of cytokines. Important cytokines that are released include IL1 and TNF-α. These and similar cytokines are necessary for the induction of adhesion molecules that attract eosinophils and other inflammatory cells into cutaneous sites. Both resident and infiltrating cells would then aggravate the inflammatory process.

ETIOLOGY

Foods

Patients with AD often have negative oral food challenges to a suspected allergen despite positive food allergen tests. Allergy skin testing for foods is a better predictor for negative reactions than positive, so interpretation should depend on history.

Food triggers for clinical atopic skin disease cannot be predicted simply by performing allergy testing. Such positive reactions must be correlated with history. At a much more complex level, double-blinded, placebo-controlled food challenges will detect clinically relevant reactions to food in AD. Using such tests, studies have demonstrated that food allergens can cause exacerbations in patients with AD. Lesions induced by a single challenge are usually transient. On the other hand, repeated challenges that are more typical of real-life exposure can result in eczematous lesions. In support of the role of food in causing AD, elimination of food allergens results in amelioration of skin disease.

Aeroallergens

Common airborne allergens such as house dust mites, animal danders, and pollens can also initiate and sustain AD. Allergen-specific IgE antibodies and allergen-specific T cells are found in patients with AD. Intranasal or endobronchial introduction of house dust mite will initiate eczema. In these patients there is a history of asthma and allergic rhinitis. Moreover, direct skin contact with inhalant allergens can also result in eczematous skin eruptions. Inhalation or contact with aeroallergens may be involved as initiating and promoting agents in the pathogenesis of AD.

Microbial Agents

Cutaneous infection is very common in AD; in one study over 50% of AD patients cultured *Staphylococcus aureus* from their skin. The organisms were endotoxin producing primarily enterotoxins A and B and toxic shock syndrome toxin-1. Specific IgE antibodies were present and directed against the staphylococcal toxins found on skin. Leung et al. have shown that exotoxins secreted by *S. aureus* can act as superantigens, which could result in persistent inflammation or exacerbations of AD.

Fungal skin infections have been associated with elevated specific IgE levels in patients with AD. Examples include lipophilic yeast *Pityrosporum ovale* and the superficial dermatophyte *Trichophyton*

rubrum. Antifungal therapy leads to clinical improvement of such patients.

Contact Reactions

Contact dermatitis has a similar appearance to other forms of chronic AD. There is a much more local response, and it is usually confined to the site of exposure.

The most common sensitizers for a contact reaction are nickel, paraphenylenediamine (PPDA), quaternium-15, neomycin, thimerosal, formaldehyde, cinnamic aldehyde, ethylenediamine, potassium dichromate, and thiuram mix. The usual sources are industrial or cosmetic. Sites involved are usually the hands and face, but generalized eruptions also occur.

Nickel allergy occurs at rates of 10–15%, making it the most prevalent cause of contact dermatitis. Nickel is ubiquitously present in diverse objects as jewelry, buttons, zippers, watchbands, some leather (from tanning), and glasses. Sensitization to nickel may occur as a result of ear piercing.

Cosmetics are a major source of allergens that may cause a contact reaction. PPDA is a pigment that is used in many dyes and inks, and is responsible for reactions to hair dyes. Quaternium-15 is a preservative that is found in many cosmetics and personal hygiene products. Patients who react to quaternium-15 may also react to formaldehyde.

Sensitization to topical medications is common, especially when applied repeatedly in small doses. Neomycin sensitization usually occurs in the clinical setting of treating ulcers with topical medications containing Thimerosal (sodium ethylmercurithiosalicylate). This is a preservative that can be present in cosmetics or topical medications, including eye drops and is a common cause for local reactions. Fragrances such as cinnamic aldehyde and cinnamic alcohol are often found in perfumes, mouthwashes, and toothpastes.

Ethylenediamine is a solubilizing component of many medications and is used in industry. Potassium dichromate is an important occupational exposure and may be present in a wide variety of materials, including chrome-plated metals, tanned leathers, and materials used in the construction industry, such as cement and plaster, glues, paints, and many others. Thiurams are another important occupational exposure and are found in the rubber industry, where they function as accelerators in the vulcanization of rubber.

There may be a reaction to sap from several types of plants. Of these, the most frequent sources are poison ivy, poison oak, and poison sumac. They produce characteristic lesions consisting of blisters in parallel lines, essentially where the vines contact the skin. Latex sensitivity is increasing in frequency, and is becoming a serious risk factor for nurses and patients with chronic latex exposure, for example, the child with spina bifida. There may be cross-sensitivity to the peel of the mango fruit and the oil from the shell of the cashew nut. Reactions to banana have also been reported in latex allergic patients.

Photocontact Dermatitis

This etiology is suggested by the clinical distribution of dermatitis, which is found only in sun-exposed areas. The face, arms, upper chest are usually prominently involved, and there is sparing of the skin under the chin, behind the ears, and of the upper eyelids. Substances that cause photocontact dermatitis require the presence of sunlight, usually in the ultraviolet band. There are two forms, phototoxic, due to sensitivity to a chemical, drug, or other substance in the presence of the invisible spectrum of sunlight, and photoallergic, which is the result of the combination of an allergy to a topical or ingested allergen and exposure to direct sunlight (Table 4-1).

Phototoxic causes are more common than photoallergic:

- Potential toxins
  - Tars
  - Dyes
  - Psoralens
- Drugs
  - Sulfonamides
  - Tetracycline
  - Thiazides
  - Phenothiazine
- Irritants
  - Fragrances
  - Sunscreen (usually to para-amino benzoic acid (PABA))

TABLE 4-1

THE ETIOLOGY OF ATOPIC DERMATITIS

Foods
 Dairy
  Eggs
  Milk
 Nuts
 Cereals
  Wheat
  Oats
 Legumes
  Peanuts
  Soybeans

Aeroallergens
 House dust mites
 Animal danders
 Pollens

Microbial Agents
 Staphylococcal toxins
 P. ovale
 T. rubrum

Contact Reactions
 Nickel
 Paraphenylenediamine (PPDA)
 Quaternium-15
 Neomycin
 Thimerosal
 Formaldehyde
 Cinnamic aldehyde
 Ethylenediamine
 Potassium dichromate

Photocontact Dermatitis
 Potential toxins
  Tars
  Dyes
  Psoralens
 Drugs
  Sulfonamides
  Tetracycline
  Thiazides
  Phenothiazine
 Irritants
  Fragrances
  Sunscreen (usually to para-amino benzoic acid (PABA))

Note: Further detail on these causes is given in the text.

CLINICAL

AD is a description of a clinical pattern that has to include the exposure history, and there are no pathognomonic skin lesions or unique laboratory parameters. In general, the principal clinical features are severe pruritus (pruritus is essential for the diagnosis of AD; there is a reduced threshold for pruritus), a chronically relapsing course, morphology in keeping with acute or chronic phase of the disease and distribution of the skin lesions that suggest the etiology, e.g., the patient's hands in a cosmetic or contact reaction, or areas that are easy to scratch in eczema. There is usually a history of atopic disease, and the presence of AD may be predictive of other atopic diseases, such as asthma.

Patients may exhibit an abnormal wheal and flare response. The usual response to scratching the skin results in blanching briefly, followed by reddening of the scratch and the formation of a wheal and surrounding flare. In AD, there is a prolonged white blanching phase, and the wheal and flare may not occur or may occur later in an incomplete way.

There are three stages: acute, subacute, and chronic.

Acute

Acute AD is characterized by intensely pruritic, erythematous papules. There are usually moderate to severe excoriations, vesiculations, and serous exudate. Secondary infection with impetigo may develop from scratching.

Subacute

Subacute AD is only slightly different from acute clinically, with more scaling noted.

Chronic

Chronic AD is the more typical appearance that is associated with AD and eczema. It is characterized by thickened skin with lichenification (accentuated markings) and fibrotic papules accompanied by anhydrosis (dry skin).

Pattern

The usual pattern of AD is that it is found in sites that are easy to scratch or at the site of contact with the irritant or allergen. In older children and adults, the lesions occur in the flexor aspects of arms and legs, especially in the popliteal and antecubital fossa. During infancy, AD involves primarily the face, scalp, and extensor surfaces of the extremities, since these are areas that the infant can scratch by rubbing against sheets or clothing. The diaper area is usually spared. Involvement in the perineal area suggests a contact reaction to an irritant. Secondary infection with staphylococcus or Candida species is not uncommon in the diaper area when it is involved.

Diagnostic Criteria

A set of diagnostic criteria published by the United Kingdom's Working Party had a high sensitivity of 85% and a specificity of 96%. The basis of this tool is itchy skin plus three or more of the following:

- Primary criteria
  - History of flexural dermatitis
  - A history of asthma or hay fever
- Generalized dry skin
- Onset of rash under the age of 2 years
- Secondary criteria
- Less reliable secondary criteria include the following:
  - Keratosis pilaris
  - Xerosis
  - Orbital pigmentation
  - Fine hair
  - Extensor dermatitis

Complications

Infection

Because of immune abnormalities seen in AD, these patients are at risk of infection. The T-cell-associated cytokine abnormalities that are often found can reduce the regulation of viral infections. The range of infections includes bacterial, viral, and fungal. In the majority of patients (>90%) with AD, *S. aureus* can be cultured from the skin. This is in marked contrast with subjects with normal skin, where only 5% have a positive culture. Patients may develop pustules or impetigo, but invasive disease is rare and should suggest an immune defect, such as hyper IgE syndrome. Because of the high frequency of positive skin cultures, patients with moderate to severe AD may benefit from a combination of antibiotic and topical steroids. Viral infections often complicate AD. These include herpes simplex virus, molluscum contagiosum, and human papillomavirus.

Fungal superinfection is associated with flares of AD. For example, *T. rubrum* infections are three times more frequent in patients with AD than in controls. Another dermatophyte, *P. ovale* is associated with head and neck distribution of AD.

Ocular Complications

Bilateral *keratoconjunctivitis* is typical of AD and is often severe. Patients present with itching, burning of the eyes, accompanied by tearing, and copious mucoid discharge. There is a risk of visual impairment from corneal scarring, often preceded by eyelid dermatitis and chronic blepharitis.

Vernal conjunctivitis is a severe form of atopic conjunctivitis, bilateral recurrent and chronic involving the upper eyelid conjunctiva. The condition is most common in young African Americans and, as the name implies, occurs primarily in the spring. There is intense pruritus which is exacerbated by irritants, sunlight, or sweating. Examination of the eye reveals papillary hypertrophy or "cobblestoning" of the upper inner eyelid surface. There may be eosinophilic infiltrates present.

Keratoconus is a conical deformity of the cornea that can cause severe visual impairment. It probably results from constant rubbing of the eyes in patients with AD and allergic rhinitis. There is an increased risk of anterior subcapsular cataracts, possibly as a consequence of the trauma of rubbing (Table 4-2).

DIFFERENTIAL DIAGNOSIS

There is a broad differential of conditions that resemble AD.

TABLE 4-2

COMPLICATIONS OF ATOPIC DERMATITIS

Infection
  Bacterial
    Staphylococcus aureus
  Viral
    Herpes simplex virus
    Molluscum contagiosum
    Human papillomavirus
  Fungal
    Trichophyton rubrum
    Pityrosporum ovale

Ocular Complications
  Keratoconjunctivitis
  Vernal conjunctivitis
  Keratoconus

Note: These problems are discussed in the text.

Scabies

Scabies is caused by skin infestation by a mite and can present as a pruritic skin disease. This is possibly due to a hypersensitivity to components of the mite, known as the Id reaction. Distribution of lesions in the genital and axillary areas, the presence of linear lesions especially in the interphalangeal web spaces, and the results of skin scrapings may help distinguish scabies from AD.

Skin Malignancies

Cutaneous T-cell lymphoma should be considered in an adult without a history of childhood atopy or other atopic features. Skin lymphomas should be suspected in an adult who has eczematous dermatitis with no history of childhood eczema and without other atopic features. The diagnosis is made by biopsies from three separate sites.

Mycosis Fungoides and Sézary Syndrome

These conditions present with plaque like lesions that superficially resemble AD or nummular eczema.

Biopsy may be needed to distinguish them from other similar looking etiologies, including AD.

Dermatitis Herpetiformis

Dermatitis herpetiformis is a rare, chronic, intensely burning, pruritic vesicular skin disease. It has been associated with a subclinical gluten-sensitive enteropathy and IgA deposits in the upper dermis. The onset is in adulthood, and the condition is rare in childhood. There is a strong association with MHC antigens B8 (60%), DR3 (95%), and DQw2 (100%).

Contact Reactions

A contactant should be considered in patients whose AD does not respond to appropriate therapy. The distribution may provide clues to the etiology of the reaction. For example, dermatitis that involves the earlobes, fingers, and wrists suggests a reaction to nickel in jewelry. Involvement of hands and forearms may indicate a work related contact exposure. A careful history of possible exposure, chemicals and other work related products, cosmetics and perfumes, soaps and laundry detergents will help to determine the cause.

Patch testing requires experienced interpretation, and can pinpoint specific chemicals and proteins. The test is performed by applying chemicals on patches to the back. The test is read by the appearance of an eczematous reaction under a patch containing a substance that causes a contact reaction in the patient.

Other Less Common Conditions

Seborrheic Dermatitis

Seborrheic dermatitis is a common, chronic, inflammatory disease probably caused by the yeast *P. ovale*. Genetic and environmental factors seem to influence the onset and course of the disease. The lesions are oily, flaky skin, different from the dry, crusty lesions of AD. The condition is common in infancy and early childhood, where it occurs primarily on the scalp. If found in adults, seborrheic dermatitis tends to persist.

Nummular Eczema

This condition is eczema that appears as one or several coin-shaped plaques. They are usually found on the legs, but can occur on the dorsum of the hand. This pattern often occurs on the extremities, but may present as hand eczema. The plaques are usually confined to the backs of the hands.

Lichen Simplex Chronicus

This condition is the result of repeated scratching in the same site, as a form of tic. It is classified as circumscribed neurodermatitis. The disease is more common in adults, but may be seen in children. The areas most commonly affected are those that are conveniently reached, usually the wrists, forearms, and hands.

Immunodeficiencies

Several congenital immune defects have prominent eczema as a presenting finding (see also Immune Defects).

- Wiskott-Aldrich syndrome
- Severe combined immunodeficiency
- Hyperimmunoglobulinemia E syndrome

Metabolic Disorders

Eczema may be the presenting feature of some metabolic disorders, or a prominent finding in the disorder (Table 4-3).

- Zinc deficiency
- Pyridoxine (vitamin B6) and niacin deficiency
- Multiple carboxylase deficiency
- Phenylketonuria

DIAGNOSIS

The diagnosis of AD is made by evaluation of the disease pattern and a careful history of exposure to potential allergens, irritants and chemicals, especially industrial. The site of lesions can often be correlated with probable exposure to the etiologic agent(s). It may be difficult to link to food reactions, as there may not be a clear temporal relationship between ingestion and the development of skin lesions.

DIFFERENTIAL DIAGNOSIS OF ATOPIC DERMATITIS

Infestations
  Scabies

Skin Malignancies
  Cutaneous T-cell lymphoma
  Mycosis fungoides
  Sézary syndrome

Sensitivity
  Dermatitis herpetiformis

Contact Reactions
  Chemicals
  Cosmetics
  Perfumes
  Soaps
  Laundry detergents

Other Less Common Conditions
  Seborrheic dermatitis
  Nummular eczema
  Lichen simplex chronicus

Immunodeficiencies
  Wiskott-Aldrich syndrome
  Severe combined immunodeficiency
  Hyperimmunoglobulinemia E syndrome

Metabolic Disorders
  Zinc deficiency
  Pyridoxine (vitamin B6) and niacin deficiency
  Multiple carboxylase deficiency
  Phenylketonuria

Note: This list is explained in the text.

History

A careful history is essential to determine the pattern of disease. An increase in pruritus after eating suspected food is helpful. A common misperception is that the AD is caused by exposure to novel antigens or irritants. In fact, a novel exposure is unlikely to result in an allergic reaction, and previous exposure is necessary to initiate an atopic response.

The history of the pattern of the lesions is less helpful, but worth obtaining. Often, the rash begins at the site of exposure which may be hands, face, neck, or groin area.

An important, but neglected aspect of the history is evaluating emotional stressors and the physical environment. There is often a psychogenic element that is part of the itch-scratch cycle in AD. There may be environmental issues that can be addressed and reduce the irritant and allergenic load.

Testing

Allergy Tests

The role of in vitro and in vivo allergy tests in AD is not clear. Performing selective food tests may be useful in confirming a suspected food or indicating that it is not a problem. Allergy tests for foods have a good correlation with negative results and are predictive of the absence of a reaction to the suspected food. They are thus helpful in excluding a food as a cause of AD. On the other hand, there is a weak predictive value for positive tests. This is especially true if there is a history of the patient eating the suspected food without problems.

Food Challenge

If it is feasible, suspected food allergies should be confirmed by double-blind, placebo-controlled food challenges. This is a tedious and potentially dangerous procedure that should be performed only by trained physicians in a hospital setting. The test is performed in the fasting state, and the suspected foods are added by opaque capsule. A placebo is used. The least suspect foods are challenged first. Using food challenge, the most frequent foods (close to 90%) associated with AD are milk, peanut, egg, soy, wheat, and fish. Avoidance of foods is difficult, but in conditions where the suspected food is completely excluded from the diet, clinical improvement is seen. This response can be used as a diagnostic tool, if the patient can avoid the suspected food.

Food Diary

A food diary is also useful. The patient records all foods eaten and annotates the diary with indications of food reactions. A pattern will emerge that can indicate foods that trigger AD. Unfortunately, the diary is seldom kept accurately.

Photopatch Test

The photopatch test is a modification of the usual patch test that is useful in diagnosing photocontact dermatitis. A duplicated patch test is placed on the back and both sets are kept covered. After 48 hours, one set is exposed to ultraviolet light and covered again. After a further 48 hours, the test is read. The test is read at 48 and 96 hours. The effect of ultraviolet exposure is assessed by comparing the exposed to unexposed test. A test patch with eczema only on the exposed side indicates a photosensitive reaction due to that allergen.

MANAGEMENT

As with most chronic diseases, the most important aspect of therapy is education of the patient and parents. Patients should especially understand that AD is chronic, and needs ongoing therapy to maintain control.

Skin Hydration

Atopic skin is very dry and demonstrates enhanced water loss that is aggravated by decreased water binding in the skin. Hydration can be restored by bathing for 15–20 minutes in lukewarm water and then applying a skin cream on lotion to retain the moisture. A facecloth soaked in warm water may be effective for the face and neck area. Oatmeal and baking soda are soothing when added to the water, but do not increase moisture uptake. Baths should not be prolonged, and bubble bath and liquid soap should not be used as these are often more irritating than bar soaps. The patient should only partly dry the skin and add lotion or skin cream. Showers may be preferable for routine and daily use. If hydrating measures are not taken within a few minutes of the bath or shower, evaporation will result in further drying and irritation. Having the parents and patients understand hydration techniques will make it easier for them to control the AD.

Moisturizers and Occlusives

The use of moisturizing agents is the cornerstone of managing AD. In more severe cases, lotions and creams may be drying, and ointments should be used. Initial hydration therapy is essential for effective use of ointments.

Emollients

Emollients help restore and preserve the skin barrier especially when combined with prior hydration therapy, and can result in a decreased need for topical corticosteroids. Moisturizers can be prepared as lotions, creams, and ointments. Lotions contain more water than creams and may have alcohols. For this reason they may be more drying than ointments. It is important to use preparations that do not have perfumes or preservatives. Eucerin, Lubriderm, Keri, and Vaseline Petroleum Jelly are useful brands.

Overnight Hydration

Wet dressings can be used to potentiate steroid therapy. This technique combines prolonged hydration and occlusion with an effective barrier to the patient scratching. The use with a lower potency steroid increases absorption of the steroid. Wet pajamas or long underwear are used with dry pajamas or sweat suit covering them. Wet tube socks under dry socks are useful for hands and feet. An alternative technique is to use wet gauze bandages under dry. Care must be taken not to overuse wet dressings, which can lead to infection, maceration of the skin or even decreased core temperature. The best use is at bedtime.

Corticosteroids

Topical corticosteroids have a dual action in the skin. They are keratolytic and reduce the thickness of the hyperkeratotic skin in AD making it easier to hydrate the skin. Steroids also have a key effect in reducing inflammation and vascular permeability. Potency of the topical skin steroids is measured by the ability to decrease vascular leak. These effects are potent at reducing pruritus in AD. There are seven levels of potency in topical steroids, with one the most potent and seven the least. (See Dermatologic Preparations in the chapter on Therapy for details and examples of each category.) The least potent topical corticosteroid that is effective should be used. High potency steroids should never be used in the groin area or on the face as they can cause significant thinning of the skin and breakdown. Children may absorb significant quantities of potent steroids, leading to side effects. For resistant lesions, the use of occlusive wrapping is helpful. This procedure is used on extremities, one limb per night to prevent overheating. The topical steroid is applied as an ointment and Vaseline is placed over the steroid. The limb is wrapped in a plastic wrap (Saran wrap). Gauze bandage is wrapped over the Saran wrap and left overnight. No stronger than medium potency steroids should be used for this procedure because of the risk of local atrophy and systemic effects. Choice of a particular product depends on the severity and distribution of skin lesions. Steroids should be discontinued once the inflammation has subsided. Hydration therapy should continue for an indefinite period.

Side effects include the following:

- Thinning of the skin
- Striae
- Acne
- Telangiectasias
- Bruising
- Hypopigmentation

There are several bases for topical corticosteroids, the most usual being ointments, creams, lotions, solutions, and sprays. Many solutions are drying because of the alcohol content. They are suitable for use in hairy areas and on the scalp. Ointments are the most occlusive and hydrating. Creams and lotions are easier to spread and not as messy as ointment, but are less effective and can cause itching. Patients may also itch because of reactions to the base and other chemicals in the steroid preparation, producing a contact dermatitis.

Recently, topical corticosteroids have been shown to decrease skin load of *S. aureus*.

Systemic

Systemic corticosteroids should be a last resort for patients with severe disease who are not responding to conventional therapy. The use of oral steroids should be short term to control a severe flare-up of AD or to gain control of the condition. There is a risk of rebound increase in symptoms after discontinuing the use of systemic steroids. To avoid this problem, even short courses of oral steroids should be tapered to discontinue them and topical steroid therapy should be intensified during the taper.

Antihistamines

Pruritus is the driving force behind AD and is the source of greatest irritation to the patient. It is unlikely that lesions will heal without controlling pruritus. Relieving itch results in a significant improvement in quality of life for patients with AD (see also Chapter 16).

Sedating antihistamines may be effective because of tranquilizing and sedative effects. They should be given at night to reduce daytime drowsiness. The use of a mild sedative to supplement antihistamines may be indicated in severe cases to help the patient sleep. Doxepin is a tricyclic antidepressant which has both anti-H1 and anti-H2 receptor binding affinity. It has a long half-life and a single 10–50-mg dose can be used in the evening.

Non-sedating antihistamines have a prolonged suppression effect on the cutaneous wheal and flare response. Loratadine 10 mg daily or cetirizine 10 mg twice daily have been shown to significantly reduce pruritus.

Topical antihistamines and local anesthetics should be used with care. The application of these and other potentially allergenic products to the skin carries a high risk of sensitization. Topical 5% doxepin cream has been effectively used, but reactions to topical doxepin have been reported.

Anti-Infectives

Bacterial

Secondary infection with *S. aureus* is very common in AD. In refractory cases, severe cases or in obviously infected skin, systemic antibiotic therapy with Erythromycin, a first-generation cephalosporin or semisynthetic penicillin may be necessary. First- or second-generation cephalosporins are effective and convenient alternatives. Maintenance antibiotic therapy should not be used because of the risk of emerging resistant organisms. Topical antistaphylococcal therapy (for example, mupirocin (Bactroban)) applied tid for 7–10 days may be effective for treating localized areas of involvement. Significant skin irritation can result from topical antibacterial agents.

Viral

If patients develop disseminated eczema herpeticum (Kaposi's varicelliform eruption), treatment with systemic acyclovir is usually required. Recurrent cutaneous herpetic infections can be controlled with daily prophylactic oral acyclovir.

Fungal

Dermatophyte infection can usually be controlled by topical antifungal drugs such as ketoconazole. Systemic antifungal therapy is very rarely indicated.

T-Cell Modulating Agents

Two medications that are potent modifiers of CD4 T-cell function (see also chapter on Immune Function) have recently been adapted for cutaneous use.

Tacrolimus (Protopic)

Ointment, 0.03%, 0.1%

Indicated in ages 2 years to adult

Tacrolimus primarily depresses T-lymphocyte function and has other effects to reduce immune activation including depression of release of cytokines IL3, IL4, IL5, GM-CSF, and TNF-α. It is used systemically to suppress graft rejection following organ transplantation. Because it is a very potent immune modifier, it should be used with caution. For moderate to severe eczema, Protopic can be used for 1 week beyond clearing of the lesions. Prolonged use is not recommended, and exposure to UV light should be avoided, since the combination of Protopic and UV exposure has been shown to decrease the time to tumor formation in mice. Protopic should not be used under occlusive dressings.

Untoward effects include the following:

- Herpes-Zoster infection
- Eczema herpeticum
- Skin burning
- Pruritus
- Erythema
- Skin infection
- Hyperesthesia
- Acne
- Folliculitis
- Urticaria

Pimecrolimus (Elidel)

Cream, 1%

Elidel is also indicated for short-term use in more refractory cases. The use of this agent should be reevaluated if symptoms do not resolve in 6 weeks. It should not be used with occlusive dressings. Pimecrolimus inhibits T-cell activation by blocking the transcription of early cytokines, especially IL2 and interferon gamma as well as IL4 and IL10. In addition, pimecrolimus prevents mast cell degranulation in vitro after stimulation by IgE dependent mechanisms. Untoward effects are similar to those for tacrolimus. In addition, there was an increased frequency of respiratory and skin infections in the Elidel group during clinical drug trials.

Cyclosporin A

Cyclosporin A (CsA) is an immunosuppressive drug that acts primarily on T cells in a manner similar to tacrolimus, with similar effects on cytokine production. Cyclosporin A seems to have an effect on IL5, which is involved in eosinophil chemotaxis. While a short course of oral Cyclosporin A in severe AD has demonstrated significant improvement in the condition, the risk of severe nephrotoxicity and CNS side effects preclude long-term use. Even after a short oral course, serum urea, creatinine, and bilirubin concentrations may be elevated, but normalize after discontinuing Cyclosporin A. Relapse rate of AD is high after stopping the drug.

Topical use of CsA in AD has yielded mixed results. Overall, the topical use of CsA does not seem to be effective.

Interferon-Gamma (IFN-γ)

Among the functions of IFN-γ is suppression of IgE synthesis and the shift away from Th2 type cell function toward Th1 type function. Subcutaneous treatment with a recombinant interferon-gamma reduced clinical severity of patients with AD. This effect persisted for several months after discontinuing therapy. IFN-γ has a significant side effect profile (fever, headache, rash, chills, fatigue, vomiting, nausea, myalgia, arthralgia) significantly limiting its usefulness for AD.

Tar Preparations

Crude coal tar extracts have a steroid sparing effect, mainly because of moderate anti-inflammatory properties. Concomitant use with topical steroids can be very effective in controlling AD and eliminate the need to use more potent steroids. This is particularly true of the scalp, where tar shampoos (T/Gel, Ionil-T) are helpful in controlling scalp lesions. It is also useful to apply moisturizers over tar products to decrease their skin drying effects. A product that contains a tar and moisturizer simplifies the application. An example is 5% LCD (Liquor Carbonis Detergens) in Aquaphor ointment.

A major drawback to tar preparations is staining of clothes and the odor that is associated with the products. Use at bedtime allows the patient to remove any odor by washing in the morning and limits staining. These are irritating preparations and should not be used on acutely inflamed skin because this may result in further skin irritation. Rarely, patients may exhibit photosensitivity reactions and pustular folliculitis.

Control of Aggravating Agents

Irritants

There is a wide range of irritants that aggravate atopic dermatitis. Moreover, patients with AD have a reduced threshold of reacting adversely to irritants. It is important to eliminate as many as possible. Irritants that are responsible include the following:

Detergents

Detergents are allergens and irritants that often cause significant irritation. They are not commonly primary causes of AD, but increase sensitivity to other allergens and may cause irritation and scratching. Residual laundry detergent left in clothes can be reduced by double rinsing. Powder soaps are harder to remove completely. Those without bleach are better tolerated.

Fabric Softeners

Chemical antistatic products, both as dryer sheets or liquid can be irritating and aggravate AD.

Soaps

Mild, unscented, neutral soaps should be used for bathing. These soaps are generally less drying or irritating, and less likely to induce pruritus. Examples are Dove, Neutrogena, Basis, and Oil of Olay; all should be unscented. Patients should limit bathing time. A shower is preferable to a bath for routine washing. A bath should be used for hydration therapy and bubble bath and scented oils completely avoided.

Chemicals

The patient's skin should be protected from household cleaners and chemicals by wearing protective gloves or clothing. Patients with AD have an altered skin barrier that is less resistant to irritants. Patients generally tolerate swimming, despite the chemicals used in public swimming pools. Showering immediately after is essential to remove chlorine.

Pollutants

Atmospheric pollution will aggravate skin disease, including AD, because of heavy metal and chemical content. Patients should be aware of the risks and use protective ointments.

Abrasives

Rough materials, such as wool, should not be worn against the skin. Materials that do not "breathe" such as nylon also irritate AD and should be avoided.

High or Low Temperatures

Temperatures that are very hot will aggravate skin conditions and increase pruritus. Hot water showers or baths can also increase the degree of irritation. The other extreme, cold air or water will increase itch and the severity of AD. Sun-exposed areas should be protected with a PABA free sunscreen without scents or perfumes. Prolonged sun exposure will cause drying and irritation of skin, with aggravation of symptoms.

Very high or low humidity will also aggravate AD. Patients should humidify the home in winter to reduce drying.

Allergens

Food

Where the patient has a positive allergy test and increased pruritus with eating a specific food, it should be avoided. On the other hand, extensive elimination diets are seldom justified or helpful, and are usually nutritionally unsound. This is especially true in children.

Contact

For patients who demonstrate positive skin tests to mites and mold, exposure will aggravate the AD. Control measures to reduce exposure, include environmental control measures aimed at reducing antigen load. Dust mite and mold-proof encasings should be used on pillows, mattresses, and box springs. Linen should be washed in hot water weekly, and bedroom carpeting removed. Indoor humidity levels should be reduced.

Psychosocial Factors

In many instances, there is a psychological overlay, and counseling may be helpful for those dealing with the frustrations of managing and living with AD. Relaxation, behavioral modification, and other methods may help patients with habitual scratching.

Patient Education

Adequate education about the disease is important in controlling AD. The goal should be to make the patient a partner in controlling the problem. Patients should understand the chronic nature of AD, what causes exacerbations, and what an appropriate treatment response should be. Patients and their families, especially those with severe disease, need written instructions that include the treatment plan. This plan should be reviewed and revised at every visit and the patient or parent should demonstrate understanding of the plan to help ensure a good outcome. An excellent source is the National Eczema Association for Science and Education at 1220 SW Morrison, Suite 433, Portland, OR 97205, Phone: 800-818-7546, Fax: 503-224-3363 or Web address: http://www.nationaleczema.org/.

Reliable information may also be obtained from the National Eczema Association on the Web at http://www.eczematreatmentinfo.com/National-Eczema-Association.html. This site has good information but patients need to ignore the advertisements for miracle cures.

Recalcitrant Disease

Hospitalization

Patients with severe AD who have extensive disease or who appear toxic will benefit from hospitalization. This approach serves several functions. The patient can be sedated to reduce pruritus, intensive skin care can be given with greater frequency than at home, and appropriate antibiotic therapy can be given. Often, removing the patient from the home environment with allergens and stressors will result in improvement. Hospitalizing the patient also provides an opportunity for intense education about AD. If indicated, the hospitalized patient can have a provocative challenge to identify triggers under controlled circumstances.

Ultraviolet (UV) Light Therapy

For patients whose disease is not exacerbated by sunlight and who are not fair complexioned, sun exposure in moderation may be beneficial. Sunburn and perspiring should be avoided. If a sunlamp is used at home, extreme caution should be exercised to avoid overexposure. Controlled use of narrow band UV under medical supervision is helpful for patients with acute exacerbations.

Photochemotherapy

Photochemotherapy utilizes the combination of a photosensitizing agent (psoralens) with UVA light. This approach may be helpful for the patient with severe, refractory AD, where there is failure of topical therapy and side effects are present. This is potentially very toxic therapy, and should only be used by physicians trained in the use of these agents. Short-term adverse effects are erythema, pruritus, and pigmentation. Long-term adverse effects are serious and include premature skin aging and cutaneous malignancies.

This is an effective form of therapy in children with disease severe enough to cause growth retardation. However, children have a high risk of cutaneous malignancies with psoralen therapy.

Potential Therapy

Allergen desensitization. This approach has been tried in uncontrolled and controlled double-blinded trials. The results are generally disappointing. Notable trials have used *Dermatophagoides pteronyssinus* extract, without any clear benefit. An interesting approach is to administer immune complexes consisting of allergen + antibody. Studies have shown early promise. Allergen desensitization is not recommended for food allergies.

ESSENTIAL FATTY ACIDS

Early studies have shown conflicting results. This approach is based on data indicating that there are abnormalities of essential fatty acid metabolism in AD.

ANTICYTOKINE OR CYTOKINE RECEPTOR THERAPY

Theoretically, blocking IL5 or IL4 would improve atopic disease. While early data indicate a reduction in eosinophils, they have not translated into clinical improvement.

PHOSPHODIESTERASE INHIBITORS

Early studies have shown promise with topical application.

Suggested Reading

Akhavan, A. and S. R. Cohen (2003). The relationship between atopic dermatitis and contact dermatitis. *Clin Dermatol* **21**(2): 158–62.

Antezana, M. and F. Parker (2003). Occupational contact dermatitis. *Immunol Allergy Clin North Am* **23**(2): 269–90; vii.

Blauvelt, A., S. T. Hwang, et al. (2003). 11. Allergic and immunologic diseases of the skin. *J Allergy Clin Immunol* **111**(Suppl. 2): S560–70.

Boguniewicz, M. and D. Y. Leung (2001). Pathophysiologic mechanisms in atopic dermatitis. *Semin Cutan Med Surg* **20**(4): 217–25.

Bradley, M., C. Soderhall, et al. (2002). Susceptibility loci for atopic dermatitis on chromosomes 3, 13, 15, 17 and 18 in a Swedish population. *Hum Mol Genet* **11**(13): 1539–48.

Brook, I., E. H. Frazier, et al. (1996). Microbiology of infected atopic dermatitis. *Int J Dermatol* **35**(11): 791–3.

Dawe, R. S. (2003). Ultraviolet A1 phototherapy. *Br J Dermatol* **148**(4): 626–37.

Granlund, H. (2002). Treatment of childhood eczema. *Paediatr Drugs* **4**(11): 729–35.

Kang, K. and S. R. Stevens (2003). Pathophysiology of atopic dermatitis. *Clin Dermatol* **21**(2): 116–21.

Kristal, L. and P. A. Klein (2000). Atopic dermatitis in infants and children. An update. *Pediatr Clin North Am* **47**(4): 877–95.

Leung, A. K. and K. A. Barber (2003). Managing childhood atopic dermatitis. *Adv Ther* **20**(3): 129–37.

Phelps, R. G., M. K. Miller, et al. (2003). The varieties of "eczema": clinicopathologic correlation. *Clin Dermatol* **21**(2): 95–100.

Stander, S. and M. Steinhoff (2002). Pathophysiology of pruritus in atopic dermatitis: an overview. *Exp Dermatol* **11**(1): 12–24.

5

ALLERGIC RHINITIS

Allergic rhinitis is a common disorder that affects approximately 20% of the general population. Allergic rhinitis embodies the most typical presentation features of allergies. The condition can range from almost trivial to severe.

USUAL CLINICAL FEATURES

General

Allergies may present at any age, but are more frequent in childhood.

There is often a seasonal pattern. In climates with distinct seasons, spring is associated with tree pollen, summer with grass, and fall with weed pollens.

The most usual presenting symptoms are spasms of sneezing accompanied by nasal and ocular itch.

Patients usually present with seasonal symptoms, more typically outdoors than indoors. The seasons that are involved and most frequently reported are fall and then spring.

There is a higher frequency in young children and teens, with a declining frequency into adulthood.

Symptoms

Patients most often complain of sneezing. This occurs in spasms, with parents reporting repeated bursts of sneezing. The symptom often occurs in the morning, but there is no typical pattern. The most striking symptom is pruritus, which is often regarded as a hallmark of allergies. Because of the release of vasoactive mediators during the allergic reaction, there is stimulation of fine nerve endings, which is interpreted as itch. The accumulation of interstitial fluid aggravates this sensation.

Less often, patients may complain of rhinorrhea, which is watery and persistent.

Patients may complain of chronic congestion. This is usually accompanied by snoring and even obstructive sleep apnea. This type of reaction is usually caused by a late phase allergic reaction. It tends to involve leukotrienes rather than histamine.

Physical Findings

Allergic Shiners

These typically involve the lower lid in the medial two-thirds. They are not specific for allergies, but reflect nasal venous congestion because venous drainage from this portion of the lower eyelid is into the nasal venous plexus.

Transverse Nasal Crease

This sign is indicative of the allergic salute, an upward motion on the tip of the nose that opens the alae and scratches the itch.

TABLE 5-1

KEY PRESENTING FEATURES OF ALLERGIC RHINITIS

Symptoms
  Sneezing
  Pruritus
  Rhinorrhea
  Chronic congestion
  Snoring

Physical findings
  Pale blue nasal mucosa
  Posterior pharynx
  Cobblestone appearance
  Mucus drainage in the posterior pharynx

Note: Further details are given in the text.

Adenoidal Facies

  Swelling across the nasal bridge
  Mouth breathing
  Nasal congestion
  Nasal mucosa

Nasal mucosa is often pale blue in color as a result of concomitant arteriolar and venous spasm with autonomic effects from allergy.

Posterior Pharynx

Effects of postnasal drainage may be seen: a cobblestone appearance and, less frequently, mucus drainage in the posterior pharynx.

There may be a pale, blue coloration to the pharyngeal mucosa as well (Table 5-1).

IMPORTANT HISTORY

Onset of Symptoms

Allergic reactions usually occur within 30 minutes of exposure.

Seasonal Pattern

Allergic rhinitis more often occurs in a seasonal pattern, while asthma is often perennial.

Indoor or Outdoor Symptoms

Indoor triggers, such as house dust mites and dander of furry animals, tend to cause perennial symptoms.

Outdoor allergens are more usually pollens of trees, grasses, and weeds.

Dual Symptoms

Antigens that are found indoors and outdoors, such as mold spores, are usually triggers for a combined response.

Environmental History

Type of Dwelling

- Obvious damp or mold
- Leaks
- Presence of a basement
- Type of heating/cooling—forced air systems distribute allergens throughout the house
- Presence of smokers and animals
- Wood burning fireplace
- Type of bedding

Problem Areas Include

- Feather pillows
- Unprotected mattress (lack of zippered protective cover)
- Proximity of parks and forest preserves
- Proximity of industry, heavy traffic, especially truck traffic

Family History

There often is a strong familial history of allergies and asthma. The patient will also commonly have other allergic symptoms, such as eczema or food allergies.

DIFFERENTIAL DIAGNOSIS

There are several forms of rhinitis. The following is a suggested approach to the diagnosis and management (Table 5-2).

TABLE 5-2
ALLERGIC AND OTHER CAUSES OF RHINITIS

	Sneezing and Itching	Rhinorrhea	Congestion
Allergic	++++	++	+
Infectious rhinitis	±	+++	+++
Perennial nonallergic with eosinophilia	+++	+++	+
Vasomotor	++	++++	+
Rhinitis medicamentosa	±	±	++++
Structural			
Septal anomalies	−	−	++++
Cocaine abuse	−	−	++++
Foreign body	−	+++	+++

Note: Symptoms are divided into sneezing and itch, rhinorrhea, and nasal congestion. This helps to distinguish allergic rhinitis from other similar looking conditions.

Symptoms can be grouped according to sneezing and itch, which are mainly due to histamine, and to a lesser extent, the leukotrienes. Rhinorrhea is prominent in vasomotor rhinitis and viral infections. Congestion is a feature of obstruction, whatever the cause.

EXPLANATION
OF DIFFERENTIAL DIAGNOSIS

Infectious

This is the most common nasal condition, and is usually caused by a rhinovirus. Other respiratory viruses, such as parainfluenza, influenza, adenovirus, and respiratory syncitial virus can cause similar symptoms. The predominant symptom is nasal pain and discomfort, rather than itch. Nasal secretions are often mucopurrulent.

Non-allergic Rhinitis
with Eosinophilia Syndromes (NARES)

NARES is a condition that resembles allergic rhinitis in all features, except for the presence of demonstrable allergies. Local and systemic eosinophilia is characteristic of the condition. There is a preponderance in women, especially in the third to fourth decades. The exact etiology is not known.

Vasomotor

Vasomotor rhinitis predominantly affects young males. It is caused by excess nasal cholinergic activity, and is aggravated by emotion and stress, spicy foods, and irritants. Patients present with a persistent, watery nasal discharge that is refractory to antihistamines, but responds well to anticholinergic agents, such as ipratropium bromide nasal spray (Atrovent).

Rhinitis Medicamentosa

This condition is a result of abuse by patients of topical α_1 agonists. Examples are Vicks nasal spray and Afrin, usually available as over-the-counter medications. These agents provide temporary relief by inducing vasoconstriction with reduction in edema. The effect wears off in 3–4 hours, with rebound hyperemia and edema. This cycle repeats, with progressive thickening of the nasal mucosa and dependence on the medication. Treatment requires the use of topical steroids, and avoidance of α_1 agonists.

Structural

These conditions present primarily with a sensation of obstruction. In the case of a deflected nasal septum, there is narrowing of the nasal passage. Interestingly, in patients who abuse cocaine, there is also a sensation of obstruction, despite the fact that cocaine causes nasal mucosal atrophy. Rhinorrhea is often a feature of chronic cocaine use.

Foreign Body

There are several characteristics that suggest the presence of a foreign body in the nasal passages. This is mostly a problem in children.

- Unilateral symptoms and signs
- Persistent rhinorrhea, often mucopurulent
- Obstructed airflow

EVALUATION OF RHINITIS

The main finding that distinguishes allergic rhinitis from other causes is the presence of positive allergy tests. Serum IgE levels are not very useful in the detection of allergies. There is not a good correlation with clinical atopy, although high levels are suggestive. Total IgE levels are not specific and do not add meaningful information (Table 5-3).

Crobach et al. demonstrated that finding nasal eosinophilia (>10% eosinophils) indicated

- 81% positive predictive value of the presence of allergies
- 55% negative prediction of the presence of allergies
- Little addition to good history
- Not recommended for general practice

Peripheral blood eosinophilia is nonspecific, and can indicate a large number of conditions that are not allergic. While elevated eosinophil counts are suggestive, they are not usually helpful clinically. On the other hand, nasal eosinophilia shows a good correlation with allergic rhinitis.

Nasal eosinophils are also present in NARES. A distinction from allergic rhinitis is made by the presence or absence of positive allergic testa.

COMPLICATIONS OF ALLERGIC RHINITIS

Recurrent Otitis Media—Relationship to Allergy

There is evidence that allergies contribute to recurrent otitis media.

Increased IgE in fluid in the middle ear has been noted.

Eustachian tube dysfunction correlates with seasonal variation in atopic patients.

Epistaxis

There is a 20% association with allergic rhinitis in children who present with recurrent epistaxis. This

TABLE 5-3

DIFFERENTIAL DIAGNOSIS OF ALLERGIC RHINITIS

	Allergy Testing	IgE	Eosinophils	Methacholine Challenge
Allergic	+ + + +	+ + +	+ + +	+
Infectious rhinitis	–	–	–	–
Nonallergic with eosinophilia	–	–	+ + + +	+
Vasomotor	–	–	–	–
Rhinitis medicamentosum	–	–	–	–
Structural				
Septal anomalies	–	–	–	–
Cocaine abuse	–	–	–	–
Foreign body	–	–	–	–

Note: Differential diagnosis depends primarily on allergy tests. Circulating IgE, the presence of eosinophils and a positive methacholine challenge are also useful. Further details are given in the text.

TABLE 5-4

THE FREQUENCY OF EPISTAXIS IN ALLERGIC
RHINITIS

Symptoms	Skin Tests	Epistaxis (%)
Positive	Positive	20.2
Positive	Negative	9.9
Negative	Positive	3.4
Negative	Negative	2.1

Note: The frequency is increased tenfold compared to patients
without symptoms or a positive allergy skin test. Children who
had a positive history but negative skin tests were five times
more likely to have epistaxis. However, those with a positive skin
test but negative history were identical to controls.

association is significantly different from nonallergic children (Table 5-4).

In the above study, 577 children in an allergy
clinic were stratified by history of allergies and
allergy skin tests. There was a tenfold greater frequency of epistaxis in children with a positive
history and positive skin tests than those who were
negative for both. Those who were positive for
history only were five times more likely to give a
history of epistaxis, while those who were positive
for skin test only did not differ from controls.

Nasal Polyps and Allergies

Polyps are rare in patients with uncomplicated
allergic rhinitis.

Polyps are a rare event in children and their
presence should suggest cystic fibrosis. The average frequencies of nasal polyps in different groups
is given in Table 5-5.

TABLE 5-5

AVERAGE INCIDENCE OF POLYPS IN DIFFERENT
DEMOGRAPHIC GROUPS AND DISEASES

Asthma	32%
Allergic rhinitis	5%
Male:female	3:1
Aspirin	5%
Children	0.5%
Cystic fibrosis	40–70%

Sinusitis

There appears to be an increased frequency of sinusitis, possibly related to chronic meatal occlusion.

Cells involved in the allergic pathway may be
found in the sinus cavity in these patients.

ALLERGIC CONJUNCTIVITIS

Conjunctivitis is a frequent manifestation of exposure to airborne or contact allergens.

Clinical Features

- Itch
- Reddened conjunctiva
- Cobblestone appearance especially on the
  palpebral conjunctiva
- A seasonal pattern is common

Differential

Infectious Conjunctivitis

Allergy is usually symmetrical, while infectious
conjunctivitis is not.

A purulent discharge may be present, and
patients complain of sticky secretions that cause their
eyelids to adhere in the morning.

Vernal Conjunctivitis

This is a condition that occurs predominantly in the
spring, in the Southeast of the United States and
mostly among African Americans. The precise cause
is not known, but there is believed to be an atopic
basis. The disease is distinguished by the presence of
accretions of eosinophils on the bulbar conjunctiva.
These are known as Tranta's spots. They may occur
at the limbus of the cornea, putting the patient at risk
for encroachment onto the cornea with possible
blindness.

THERAPY OF ALLERGIC RHINITIS

Therapeutic options include the use of medications
that block histamine and leukotrienes and that

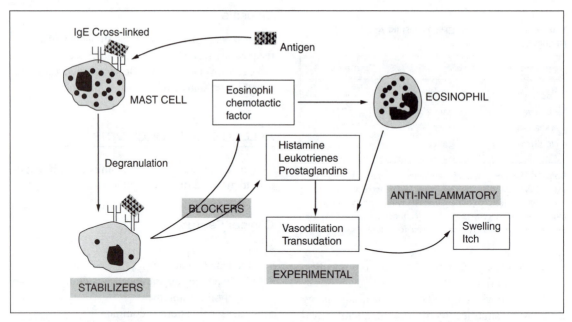

FIGURE   5 - 1

BASIC CASCADE OF THE IMMUNE RESPONSE THAT PRODUCES AN ALLERGIC REACTION (DISCUSSED IN CHAP. 2, FIGURE 2-1).

The major groups of medications used in the therapy of allergic rhinitis and the site of their action are shown in the grey boxes in this figure.

reduce inflammation. There are mast cell stabilizing drugs that prevent activation of the allergic cascade (Figure 5-1, Table 5-6).

TREATMENT STRATEGIES

Allergic Rhinitis

Environmental control and allergen avoidance
Non-sedating antihistamines
Topical antihistamines/anticholinergic
Nasal cromolyn
Nasal steroids
Immunotherapy

Allergic Conjunctivitis

Environmental control
Nonsedating antihistamines

Topical antihistamines
Topical mast cell stabilizers
Nasal steroids
Immunotherapy

TABLE   5 - 6

SITE OF ACTION OF ALLERGY MEDICATIONS

Site of action	Medication
Blockers	Antihistamines
	Leukotriene blockers
	Anticholinergic
Anti-inflammatory	Topical steroids
Stabilizers	Cromolyn
	Nedocromil
	Olopatadine
	Ketotifen

Note: Details of their use are given in Chap. 14—Medications and Therapeutic Methods. The position in the allergy cascade that each of these medications occupies is shown on Figure 5-1.

USE OF IMMUNOTHERAPY IN ALLERGIC RHINOCONJUNCTIVITIS

Immunotherapy is also discussed in Chap.16.

PATIENT SELECTION

Specifically, in allergic rhinitis, the use of immunotherapy should be reserved for patients with

> Severe, incapacitating symptoms
> Clearly identifiable antigen(s)
> History
> Allergy testing

The history should correlate with the allergy testing or other means of antigen identification. A patient with a positive test to ragweed should have symptoms in the fall.

Immunotherapy should be reserved for patients who have a situation where

- Antigens cannot be avoided
  - Industrial situations
  - Refusal to remove animals
  - Pollen allergy
- Treatment failure
  - Lack of response to adequate pharmacotherapy
  - Side effects of medication

METHOD

For ideal results, the fewest number of antigens possible should be used. Only allergens that give the strongest positive tests should be used.

The patient is started at a 1/200,000 dilution, and the dose is increased weekly as tolerated.

The incidence of side effects is small, but the potential remains. The patient must be observed for 30 minutes following injection. The usual course of injections is over 5–6 years. The frequency of injections is reduced as the patient's tolerance of higher concentrations improves.

Suggested reading

Baroody, F. M. (2003). Allergic rhinitis: broader disease effects and implications for management. *Otolaryngol Head Neck Surg* **128**(5): 616–31.

Bhalla, P. L. (2003). Genetic engineering of pollen allergens for hayfever immunotherapy. *Expert Rev Vaccines* **2**(1): 75–84.

Bousquet, J., P. van Cauwenberge, et al. (2002). Allergic rhinitis and its impact on asthma. In collaboration with the World Health Organization. Executive summary of the workshop report. 7–10 December 1999, Geneva, Switzerland. *Allergy* **57**(9): 841–55.

Durham, S. R. and S. Walker (2000). Immunotherapy for hayfever. *Chem Immunol* **78**: 199–208.

Lin, H. and T. B. Casale (2002). Treatment of allergic asthma. *Am J Med* **113**(Suppl. 9A): 8S–16S.

Moverare, R. (2003). Immunological mechanisms of specific immunotherapy with pollen vaccines: implications for diagnostics and the development of improved vaccination strategies. *Expert Rev Vaccines* **2**(1): 85–97.

Mucha, S. M. and F. M. Baroody (2003). Relationships between atopy and bacterial infections. *Curr Allergy Asthma Rep* **3**(3): 232–7.

Novak, N. and T. Bieber (2003). Allergic and nonallergic forms of atopic diseases. *J Allergy Clin Immunol* **112**(2): 252–62.

Settipane, R. A. (2003). Rhinitis: a dose of epidemiological reality. *Allergy Asthma Proc* **24**(3): 147–54.

Togias, A. (2003). Rhinitis and asthma: evidence for respiratory system integration. *J Allergy Clin Immunol* **111**(6): 1171–83; quiz 1184.

Van Cauwenberge, P. (2002). Advances in allergy management. *Allergy* **57**(Suppl. 75): 29–36.

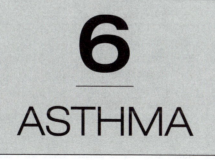

6

ASTHMA

DEFINITION

There are three main components that define asthma.

Asthma is a *reversible, recurrent obstructive* lung disease. In chronic asthma, reversibility may be only partial.

NEW UNDERSTANDING IN PATHOPHYSIOLOGY

There has been an increase in the understanding of the pathophysiology of asthma over the past several years that has formed the basis of improved therapy and recognition of the disease. A key to the development of clinical asthma is the concept of airway hyperactivity.

Basis for Airway Hyperactivity

Genetic Predisposition

There are descriptions of several alleles that are associated with an increased risk of developing asthma. There is a stronger association with asthma for those links that also correlate with increased IgE production. An example is a locus on the long arm of chromosome 11 that is linked to asthma and allergies. There is also increased association of a locus on chromosome 5 (5q31-q33) that may be linked to dust mite sensitivity and have a higher frequency in African Americans.

Loci on chromosome 8 (8p23) have similar associations. There appears to be a greater linkage with Whites on chromosomes 2q21 and 13q32-q34.

It is evident that asthma is a result of a mass effect of several small genetic errors, and harder to predict than a single major mutation.

In general, the pattern of asthma inheritance is polygenic.

Cellular (Inflammatory) Component

It is now widely accepted that the major mechanism underlying asthma is chronic peribronchial inflammation. A large number of cells are involved in the inflammation of asthma. They share several mediators and produce others that are unique for a cell type. Predominant cells are eosinophils and neutrophils. The net effect of mediator release is goblet cell hypertrophy with an increase in mucus production, increase in smooth muscle tone with airway narrowing, endothelial damage, and an infiltrate of eosinophils and neutrophils. There is also an increase in lymphocytes. Specific mediators, such as eosinophil cationic protein, cause considerable damage to endothelium and epithelium (Table 6-1, Figure 6-1).

TABLE 6-1

COMMON INFLAMMATORY CELLS RELEASING MEDIATORS SPECIFIC FOR EACH CELL TYPE

Specific Mediators	Source	Common Mediators
Histamine	Mast cells	Leukotrienes
Major basic protein	Eosinophils	Prostaglandins
Cationic protein	Eosinophils	Interleukins
Serotonin	Platelets	Enzymes
Peroxide	Polymorphonuclear	Platelet activating factor
	Eosinophils	
Interleukins	T cells	

Note: Common inflammatory cells release mediators that are specific for each cell type, listed in the column on the left. The right hand column lists mediators that are common to all inflammatory types of cells named in the central column.

Ancillary Mechanisms

While inflammation is the most prominent of the pathophysiologic mechanisms for the development of asthma, it is not the only one.

There are numerous pathways that lead to acute and chronic narrowing of the airways.

Neurological Mechanisms

Autonomic imbalance. There is increased parasympathetic tone in asthma, resulting in an imbalance between sympathetic and parasympathetic control. This discrepancy is aggravated further by sympathetic underactivity.

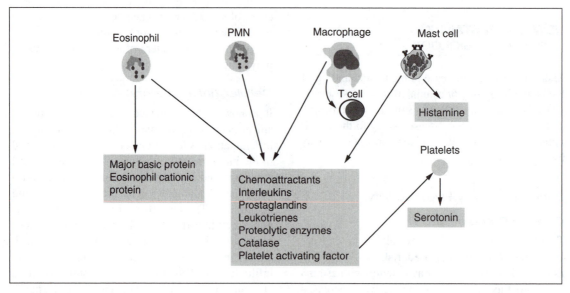

FIGURE 6-1

RANGE OF MEDIATORS THAT ARE PRODUCED BY INFLAMMATORY CELLS IN THE LUNG IN ASTHMA.

This figure complements Table 6-1. The central box lists some of the mediators that are produced by all inflammatory cells. Many cell types release unique inflammatory substances. Eosinophils produce two potent basic proteins that are destructive to cell membranes, and mast cells produce histamine. Platelet activating factor is produced by all cells and stimulates platelets to produce serotonin. PMN: polymorphonuclear cells.

Other neurogenic factors. There are several other neurogenic substances that can increase airway tone and secretions:

C afferent fibers
Substance P

Loss of Factors
Maintaining Airway Patency

Mucosa. Damage to mucosal integrity is frequent in asthma. There are several consequences to breaching the epithelial lining. First, there is a loss of smooth muscle relaxing factors, such as epithelial-derived relaxant factor and vasoactive intestinal peptide. These mediators oppose the effects of bronchocon-strictors, such as histamine and leukotrienes. With damage from eosinophil products, cationic protein for example, there is loss of mucosa surface and with it the smooth muscle relaxing factors that are produced there.

Nonadrenergic noncholinergic nervous system. The net effect of these mediators is to oppose airway constriction. They include:

Neuroendocrine
Epinephrine

Airway Changes
During an Acute Episode

An acute asthmatic episode usually follows a clearly defined pathway. The airways are not uniformly affected, resulting in unequal distribution of air and blood flow. Following exposure to a triggering agent, there is:

- Bronchoconstriction
- Mucosal edema
- Increased mucus production

Because of the large number of terminal bronchial units in the lungs, asthmatic changes do not occur uniformly throughout the lungs. As shown in Figure 6-2, initial events during an acute episode include bronchospasm, mucosal edema, and increased mucus secretion with narrowing of the bronchial lumen, which leads to obstruction to airflow on exhalation, rather than on inspiration.

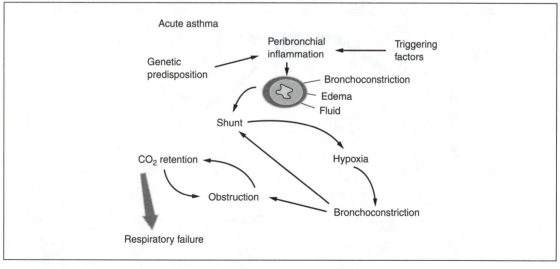

FIGURE 6-2

PATHOGENESIS OF AN ACUTE ASTHMATIC EPISODE.

There are two self-perpetuating loops. The first occurs early in the course of an acute episode, with hypoxemia based on a ventilation-perfusion mismatch. As this loop progresses, it leads into the second, with CO_2 retention. If this second loop is not interrupted, the patient is at serious risk of progressing to respiratory failure.

TABLE 6-2

A COMPARISON OF THE EARLY AND LATE PHASES OF ASTHMA

Phase	Associations	Onset
Early	Histamine and cholinergic mediation IgE receptors Self-limited	Immediate to 30 minutes
Late	Mast cells/histamine IgE dependent Increased morbidity and mortality	4–6 hours

Note: This table complements Figure 6-3.

This is not a uniform process throughout the lungs. As a result, there are areas that are overdistended because of air trapping, but have poor blood supply because of stretching of blood vessels. Other areas are collapsed because of more complete obstruction. These areas have an increased blood supply. This pattern results in a ventilation-perfusion ($\dot{V}/\dot{Q}$) mismatch. Normally $\dot{V}/\dot{Q} = 1$, and deviations from this ratio can result in hypoxemia.

The initial event in an acute asthmatic episode is hypoxemia, which leads to tachypnea and tachy-cardia. The implication is that patients with an acute asthmatic presentation who have increased heart and respiratory rate are probably hypoxemic. This pattern develops into a cycle with hypoxemia increasing bronchospasm, which in turn causes an increase in hypoxia. As the bronchospasm worsens, the patients start to trap air and CO. If treatment is not instituted at this stage, the process is likely to progress inexorably to respiratory failure.

The increase in airway secretions is primarily an increase in the water phase of mucus. This

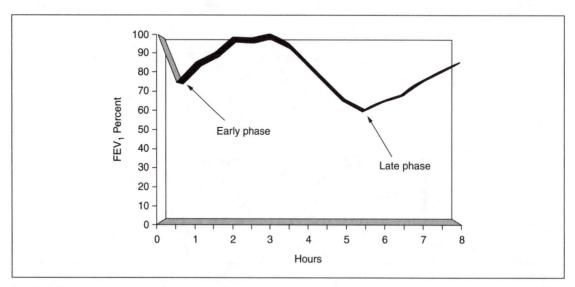

FIGURE 6-3

REPRESENTATION OF EARLY AND LATE PHASE ASTHMA.

The early phase is of short duration, and has a rapid onset. The late phase is long lasting and more severe with an onset 4–6 hours after exposure to the antigen. This phenomenon is described further in the text. FEV1: forced expiratory volume in 1 second; a measure of airway obstruction.

results in lifting of the mucin blanket above the cilia of bronchial epithelium. The patient will develop a harsh, dry cough that is characteristic of asthma because they are unable to mobilize the increased secretions (Figure 6-2).

Early and Late Phase Reactions in Asthma

An important pathologic event is the biphasic response of the airways. The early phase is the result of bronchospasm, and onset is within 30 minutes. This phase is typically seen clinically as the acute asthma episode, and may resolve spontaneously over 2–3 hours.

The late phase has an onset about 6 hours after the initial exposure, and lasts 2–4 days. This phase is associated with infiltration into the peribronchial space by eosinophils and neutrophils and has been linked clinically with morbidity and mortality in asthma. This pattern gives rise to a clinical problem, as a patient who is having a late phase reaction may give the appearance of initial improvement, with subsequent development of more severe airway obstruction as the late phase develops (Table 6-2, Figure 6-3).

Concept of Early Onset of Asthma

The concept of onset of allergies and asthma in childhood, also known as the Hygiene Hypothesis is presented in Chap. 3.

CLINICAL EVALUATION

History

The clinical presentation of asthma varies widely, especially in children. A careful history usually provides the key to diagnosis. The essential features are a recurrent pattern of respiratory symptoms that occur in response to defined triggers such as upper respiratory tract infections and exercise (Table 6-3). Often, the key symptom in children is cough, which follows the pattern of asthma and occurs at night and with exposure to allergens. Key features in the history are as follows:

TABLE 6-3

TRIGGERING AGENTS FOR AN ACUTE ASTHMATIC EPISODE

Group	Examples
Infections	Viral
	Upper respiratory
Allergens	Mites, mold, pollens, animal dander
Pollutants	Particulate, gaseous
Irritants	Scents, perfumes
Cold	Cold air
Exercise	Sustained > static

Note: These factors act on an airway that is primed by peri-bronchial inflammation.

Onset and History of Disease

Useful features in the history are the age at onset of the condition and the precipitating triggers. This should include when symptoms occur, day or night, and whether there is a seasonal incidence. There is no predictive value in the age of onset of symptoms. However, several investigators (Martinez) have noted with early onset of asthma symptoms that there is an increased risk of ongoing symptoms after the age of 5–6 where there is a strong family history of asthma and allergies and the child has evidence of allergies.

Typical Episode

The onset of an episode of asthma can be abrupt or gradually increase in intensity. In children, cough is often the only manifestation. The patient may complain of chest pain, tightness, or difficulty breathing. Asthma episodes are more frequent at night, especially in the early morning hours. The response to medication, especially bronchodilators, should be noted.

Associated Conditions

It is not infrequent to have comorbid conditions accompany asthma. Common examples that aggravate asthma and can render the patient refractory to medication, especially steroids are as follows:

Chronic sinus disease. There is strong evidence that recurrent or chronic sinus disease aggravates airway reactivity.

Gastroesophageal reflux. Studies have shown that the presence of acid in the lower esophagus increases lower airway resistance and can initiate or worsen an acute asthmatic episode. Reflux only needs to be into the lower portion of the esophagus to worsen asthma, and may be completely silent. It should be considered in any patient with refractory symptoms.

Pattern

A review of the pattern of symptoms often will give an indication of the triggers of an acute asthmatic episode. Where the diagnosis is not clear, as with a child with chronic cough, an association of the patient's symptoms with the common triggers of asthma should increase the level of suspicion that asthma is present.

Useful Questions Include

Frequency of interference with activities

Is the patient able to exercise or participate in sports activities?
Can the child keep up with peers?
How much work or school is missed?
How often does the parent miss work because the child is ill?

Frequency of interference with sleep. Nocturnal cough is often seen in children. Nocturnal symptoms that occur more often than twice per month indicate that the patient needs controlling medications.

Number of ER visits. Ideal therapy of asthma is preventative and not by crisis. Frequent ER visits indicate that there is poor control of the disease.

Number of hospitalizations

Number of days missed from school. This is often a difficult number to obtain. Using a defined period, such as the previous 3 months can help the parent's recall.

The following questions imply very severe disease:

Have you ever been on a ventilator?
Have you ever lost consciousness?

Perception of Severity

The patient's or parent's assessment of how severe the asthma is can be helpful in determining control. Often, patients have very poor self-evaluation. This problem is usually seen in more severe asthmatics due to a loss of perception of dyspnea. There may be a similar lack of awareness that the patient is having difficulty breathing even among less severe patients.

Precipitating Factors

The so-called "types" of asthma actually represent the effects of a variety of triggering agents in an airway primed by underlying inflammation.

Examples are shown in Table 6-3 and described below.

Infections

Respiratory tract viral infections are the major cause of acute episodes of asthma, especially in children. These can affect either upper or lower respiratory tract.

Allergens

A wide variety of allergens, such as animal dander, mold, dust mites, cockroach antigen and pollen of trees, grasses or weeds are major triggers for acute asthmatic episodes in sensitive children. Close to 80 percent of children with asthma have allergies.

Cold and Exercise

Both of these factors operate by cooling and/or drying of the bronchial mucosa. Cold air is an important bronchonstrictor.

Environment

There are numerous environmental agents that can result in an acute asthmatic episode. There are several categories that include allergens and direct airway irritants.

Industry. Many of the chemicals that are used in industry are highly irritating to the mucosa of the airway, or produce an IgE mediated response. Trimellic anhydrides produce an acute response, and can also cause IgG mediated hypersensitivity reactions, especially with prolonged, lower concentration exposure. Chemicals that contain heavy metals, especially platinum salts, also cause significant reactions. Ethylene diamine is used in the curing of rubber, and causes a strong bronchospastic and inflammatory response. Isocyanates are the product of packing materials and foam products. Many enzymes, such as occur in cleaners and detergents, are a source of respiratory distress among workers involved with the manufacture of these products.

Additionally, older working environments may have a high mold content that will affect sensitized individuals.

Parks and farms. The pollen of trees and weeds form the major allergenic load in parks. The tilling of the soil on farms encourages the growth of weeds, especially ragweed, among the crops.

Home. The major sources of triggering allergens in the home are carpeting, animals, bedding, heating and cooling ducts. Tobacco continues to be the major indoor pollutant.

Impact of Disease

On Patient

Asthma is not always evident or clearly recognized by the patient. There may be a significant impact on the patient's lifestyle, which may be accepted as normal.

On Family

A chronic disease always has a significant impact on a family that includes disruption of normal family interactions and activities such as missed vacations and frequent nights spent in an emergency room. The child with the chronic disease may receive a disproportionate amount of attention, causing resentment among other children and family members.

CLINICAL PRESENTATION

There is a wide range of presentations of asthma.

Acute

The typical acute presentation is abrupt in onset with dyspnea, increased work of breathing, cough, and breathlessness. The patient is often unable to complete a sentence without taking several breaths. Posture may indicate the degree of distress. The patient will hunch forward increasingly as distress increases, often elevating the shoulders. In extreme situations, the patient may adopt a position on hands and knees. This progressive posture allows for increased muscle action, especially by the pectoralis muscles as accessory muscles. Increasing respiratory distress is also seen in the progressive use of accessory muscles in sequence: flaring of the alae nasi, suprasternal retractions, intercostal retractions, and then subcostal retractions.

Significance of Clinical Findings in Acute Asthma

Table 6-4 indicates the significance of the usual signs and symptoms of an acute asthmatic episode. Tachypnea and tachycardia are the result of hypoxemia and are the first sign during an acute episode (Table 6-4).

Wheezing. Wheezing is very unhelpful as a sign. It only indicates that there is turbulence in the airways and does not provide information about where the obstruction is, what is causing it, or how severe the obstruction is. Patients who have severe obstruction of the airways in asthma may not have wheezing at all, as they do not move enough air to generate turbulent flow. It is much more useful to monitor airflow and the inspiration to expiration ratio for prolongation of exhalation.

TABLE 6-4

SIGNIFICANCE OF THE USUAL CLINICAL FINDINGS IN ASTHMA ARE PRESENTED IN THE RIGHT HAND COLUMN

Finding	Significance
Tachycardia	Hypoxemia
Tachypnea	Hypoxemia
Prolonged expiration	Increased obstruction
Wheezing	Unhelpful—only indicates airway turbulence and not site or severity of obstruction
Accessory muscles	Severe distress
Cyanosis	Severe $\dot{V}/\dot{Q}$ mismatch
Reduced peak flow	Severe asthma
Increased pulsus paradoxus	Severe asthma

Dangerous scenario. A 9-year-old child presents to the emergency department with a history of cough for 2 days. He is known to have asthma. Physical examination indicates mild tachypnea. Examination of the chest with tidal breathing indicates the absence of wheezing. When the child is induced to perform forceful breathing, there is fair air movement on inhalation, but on exhalation air movement is strikingly reduced. Wheezing is still not detected.

There are *two pitfalls* in this situation that can lead to a severe outcome.

First, respiration should always be assessed at maximal effort. In this case, severe airway obstruction would have been missed.

Second, focusing on wheezing could lead to missing airway obstruction that is so severe that exhalation is silent.

Pulsus paradoxus. This measurement is a difference in systolic blood pressure between inspiration and expiration. This discrepancy is usually 6–8 mmHg, The difference increases with increasing respiratory distress in proportion to the swings in plural pressure, and may be greater than 20 mmHg in severe asthma.

Nonurgent Presentation

Tiredness. Patients often complain of tiredness, chest tightness and may notice wheezing or whistling in the chest.

Cough. Cough is especially a common feature in childhood where it may be the only symptom.

The cough is frequently described as deep, wet, and non-productive, often harsh in nature. Patients will note that the cough is worse at night and on exposure to cold air. Upper respiratory tract infections are also frequent triggers.

Exercise intolerance. Aerobic exercise is particularly troublesome as it causes cooling of the airways and a change in surface tonicity. These are key factors in triggering an acute asthmatic episode.

Physical findings. Between episodes, the physical examination may not be very useful. Vital signs are normal. Cyanosis at rest and clubbing of the fingernails are not features of asthma, and their presence should suggest another disease process.

Pulmonary examination is often unremarkable between episodes. There may be a reduction in exhalation with forced expiration.

CLASSIFICATION OF ASTHMA (NHLBI GUIDELINES)

In 1992, the Heart, Lung and Blood Institute of the National Institutes of Health presented the Guidelines to the Management of Asthma in the form of the National Asthma Education and Prevention Program (NAEPP). This program was revised in 1998. A pediatric specific version and supportive literature evidence were released in 2002. The full version of the program can be seen and downloaded at http://www.nhlbi.nih.gov/guidelines/asthma/.

One very useful section of NAEPP provides a classification of asthma, shown in Table 6-5. Mild asthma is further classified as episodic or chronic.

Persistent symptoms are indicated by the criteria shown in Table 6-6.

DIAGNOSIS OF ASTHMA

The diagnosis of asthma depends to a large extent on history and the pattern of presentation, as noted above. Symptoms of chest discomfort, breathlessness, or chest pain are often associated with the usual triggers of asthma. Symptoms that wake the patient from sleep, usually in the early hours of the morning are highly suggestive of asthma. Exercise is another significant trigger, especially vigorous and aerobic activity. A history of relief with a bronchodilator is useful, since this response is the equivalent of demonstrating reversibility.

Pulmonary Function

The typical pattern seen on pulmonary function studies demonstrates airflow obstruction. There is also evidence of air trapping with an increase in residual volume. (See Chap. 11 for an essential description of pulmonary function.)

Specifically, there is a reduction in FEV1 and FEF25—75%. FVC may also be reduced as a result of air trapping, and RV would be concomitantly increased. Airway resistance is increased and conductance is reduced.

TABLE 6-5

CLASSIFICATION OF ASTHMA ACCORDING THE NAEPP, RELEASED BY THE NATIONAL HEART, LUNG AND BLOOD INSTITUTE OF THE NATIONAL INSTITUTES OF HEALTH

	Mild Intermittent	Mild Persistent	Moderate	Severe
Frequency	<2/wk	>2/wk but <1/day	>1–2/wk	Daily severe
Interval symptoms	Few	Few	Cough low grade	Continuous
Exercise tolerance	Good	Good	Diminished	Poor
Nocturnal	<2/month	>2/month	2–3/week	Considerable
Attendance	good	Good	Fair	Poor
PEFR	>80% predicted var. <20%	>80% predicted var. 20–30%	60–80% predicted var. 20–30%	<60% predicted var. >30%
Spirometry				
Obstruction	None	None	Reduced flow	Sustained
Volumes	Normal	Normal	Increased	Marked increase
Response	>15%	>15%	>15%	Incomplete
Methacholine	PC20 >20mg/mL	PC20 >20mg/mL	PC20 2–20mg/mL	PC20 <2mg/mL
Response to therapy	Good	Good	Slower	Poor/incomplete

Note: From a clinical perspective, the most significant distinction in the classification is between episodic and persistent symptoms. Patients who have persistent symptoms require controller therapy, while those with intermittent symptoms can usually take a bronchodilator as needed. (See chapter 14.)

The diagnosis of asthma is based on reversal of obstruction, and is defined by a greater than 12% increase in FEV1 following the use of a bronchodilator. Other parameters should also reverse, to varying degrees. Air trapping seems to be less responsive to a bronchodilator, but RV will usually decrease with albuterol.

Peak flow monitoring is recommended in the NAEPP. A peak flow meter is a simple spring loaded

TABLE 6-6

THE ESSENTIAL CRITERIA DERIVED FROM NAEPP THAT INDICATE THAT A PATIENT HAS PERSISTENT ASTHMA SYMPTOMS AND NEEDS CONTROLLER MEDICATION

Criterion	Frequency
Use of rescue medication	>2x/week
Nocturnal symptoms	>2x/month
Oral corticosteroids	>2x/year
Number of reliever canisters	>1/year

device that measures the most rapid flow of air during a forced expiration. The rate is expressed in liters per minute and is reflective of large to medium airway patency. The test is effort dependent, so that the result is usually recorded as the best of three attempts. NAEPP recommends the use of an inverted traffic light system. There are three zones: green, yellow, and red. These values are based on predicted values or personal best, shown in Table 6-7.

Figure 6-4 is an algorithm of the management of the acute episode for the patient at home. It is based on NAEPP. In an acute asthmatic episode, the most important approach is to have the patient receive a rescue medication as quickly as possible.

Two approaches are useful where the diagnosis is not clear, and pulmonary function is not diagnostic, peak flow monitoring and airway challenge.

Peak Flow Monitoring

The less technological approach is to have the patient monitor peak flow for 2–3 weeks tid and record the results. The patient should use a bronchodilator when PF is less than 80% of predicted.

TABLE 6-7

RESPONSE TO PEAK FLOW MEASUREMENTS

Zone	Range	Response
Green	>80% predicted	No therapy is indicated
Yellow	50–80% predicted	Use rescue medication, repeat in 30 minutes if no response Contact MD, may need steroids orally If responds, repeat rescue in 2 hours and continue regular medications
Red	<50% predicted	Take rescue medication, start steroid, if responds, repeat in 20–30 minutes To see MD as soon as possible If no response, take another treatment and seek immediate medical care

Note: The patient can base the zones on predicted values or on personal best. Since many asthmatics never attain predicted values, personal best is more meaningful. These responses are used as the basis for a written action plan.

The advantage of this approach is that it measures real world stresses such as activities and allergen exposure and the patient's pulmonary response. A pattern of reduced peak flow that responds to a bronchodilator is diagnostic of asthma.

Airway Challenge

The second approach is to challenge the patient's airway, using pulmonary function before and after the challenge as a measure of response. The "gold standard" is a challenge with methacholine, an

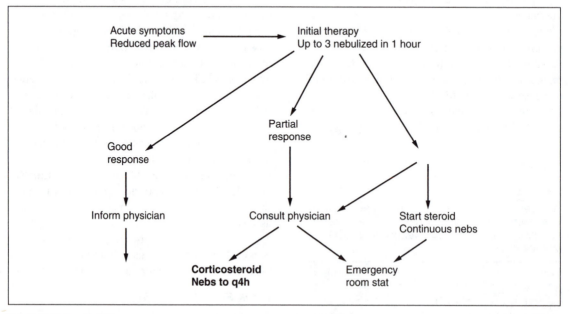

FIGURE 6-4

ALGORITHM INDICATING THE RESPONSE OF AN ASTHMATIC PATIENT HAVING AN ACUTE EPISODE AT HOME.

acetylcholine analog. The endpoint is a reduction in FEV1 by 20%, expressed as the concentration that is needed to achieve this fall. This level is termed the PC20. Inhalation challenges can also be performed using cold air, specific allergens and hypertonic saline. The patient can be physically challenged, using a treadmill or bicycle ergometer. In an exercise challenge, the endpoint is a 20% reduction in FEV1.

Figure 6-5 illustrates an algorithm to determine the presence of asthma based on the NAEPP. A pulmonary function study will either show obstruction or not. Reversal of FEV1 by more than 12% indicates asthma. Partial reversal may indicate chronic asthma, with a fixed component. If the obstruction does not reverse, the patient can be given a bronchodilator for 2 weeks and then repeat the pulmonary function. If no initial obstruction is noted, the patient should measure and record peak flow for 2 weeks. If the pattern over that period demonstrates

obstruction, then reversibility should be assessed. If no obstruction is noted (or as an alternative procedure) a challenge test can be administered. If positive, this indicates the presence of asthma, and if negative, another diagnosis should be sought.

Radiology

X Ray Chest

An x ray of the chest is probably the most requested and least helpful study in asthma. The typical findings are the following:

- Hyperinflation
- Subsegmental atelectasis
- Peribronchial cuffing
- Hyperlucency of the lungs
- Narrowing of the mediastinum

These findings can resemble infiltration or pneumonia, and give no indication of the severity

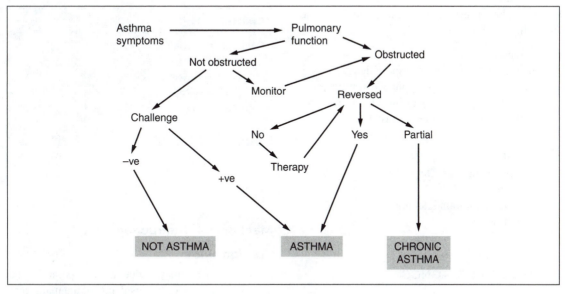

FIGURE   6 - 5

DIAGNOSTIC ALGORITHM TO DETERMINE WHETHER ASTHMA IS PRESENT OR NOT, DERIVED FROM THE NAEPP.

A pulmonary function study is used to detect the presence or absence of obstruction to airflow. If obstruction is present and reverses by >12%, asthma is present. Where there is no response, the patient will be given therapy and then reevaluated. See the text for details of this approach.

of the asthma. Since the pulmonary findings of asthma may not be uniform throughout the lungs, an incorrect conclusion may be drawn from the radiograph.

A radiographic examination of the chest should be performed on a child with new onset wheeze and asthma symptoms. Subsequently, the test is useful for answering specific questions, such as whether a febrile patient with acute asthmatic symptoms has pneumonia, or a patient who suddenly deteriorates has a pneumothorax. A chest x ray is otherwise not useful in acute asthma.

CT Scan

CAT scan is indicated to exclude bronchiectasis, especially associated with allergic bronchopulmonary aspergillosis (ABPA).

ABPA. ABPA is a complication in steroid dependent asthmatics where there is a chronic infiltration of the proximal airways by aspergillus species. These patients are also allergic to aspergillus, and have chronic airway inflammation and asthma. The criteria for diagnosis include the following:

- Refractory asthma
- Positive prick skin test to aspergillus
- The presence of fungal hyphae in sputum
- Circulating IgG antiaspergillus antibodies
- Fusiform (central) bronchiectasis

Other Studies

Allergy testing (see Chap. 12)
Sweat test
Quantitative immunoglobulins
Bronchoscopy

DIFFERENTIAL DIAGNOSIS

There is an extensive differential for the symptoms of asthma, especially in younger children. It is worth noting that several synonyms are still in use to describe an asthma pattern in infants and young children: bronchitis, wheezy bronchitis, and reactive airways disease (Table 6-8).

TABLE 6-8

DIFFERENTIAL DIAGNOSIS OF ASTHMA

Mechanical Obstruction
  Foreign body
  Chronic obstructive pulmonary disease
  Vascular rings
  Tumors
  Webs and membranes

Laryngeal Defects
  Laryngeal dysfunction
  Laryngotracheomalacia and bronchomalacia

Bronchopulmonary Dysplasia (BPD)

Infections
  Pneumonia
  Respiratory syncytial virus (RSV)
  Parainfluenza
  Adenoviruses
  Recurrent aspiration

Cardiac Disease
  Left heart failure
  Mitral valve disease

Cystic Fibrosis

Confounding Variables
  Rhinitis/sinusitis
  Gastroesophageal reflux
  Aspirin sensitivity
  Sulfite sensitivity
  Beta-blockers

Mechanical Obstruction

Foreign Body

A foreign body may lodge at any point in the bronchial tree, but usually is in one of the main stem bronchi or a first order branch. In children, parts of toys, such as wheels or eyes, and food, especially peanuts, are most frequent objects that are inhaled. In adults, loose teeth and dentures are common, with food also frequent. The most useful history is of choking; other symptoms such as cough or wheezing are not specific. Adults and older children usually aspirate foreign objects when they have altered levels of consciousness, as with drug and alcohol use, or cerebral injury or stroke. A fully alert adult may also give a history of choking on food or while eating.

Physical findings that are helpful include unequal breath sounds, unilateral wheezing, a musical pitch to the wheeze and intermittent wheezing. An important feature is the lack of a response to a bronchodilator. Chest x ray may indicate unilateral hyperinflation of one lung. If the foreign body is radiopaque, it can be seen on a plain film of the chest. Fluoroscopy will demonstrate that only one diaphragm is mobile. A more definite diagnosis can be made by CT scan or on bronchoscopy. The object can usually be removed via a bronchoscope.

Chronic Obstructive Pulmonary Disease

The key feature that distinguishes asthma and COPD is reversibility.

Vascular Rings

Vascular anomalies usually cause obstruction when they form a complete ring around a bronchus or the trachea. This is usually a diagnostic dilemma in infants and young children. Examples include a double aortic arch, aberrant subclavian artery, and compression by the innominate artery. Because the obstruction is of a large airway, there is usually wheezing on inspiration and expiration. There is no change with a bronchodilator. The diagnosis can be made by barium swallow where an indentation can be seen on the esophagus. A CT scan with infusion is more definitive, and angiography will define the abnormality. A corrective surgical procedure is usually needed.

Tumors

Masses can be in the bronchial lumen, in the wall or compressing from outside the wall. The types of tumors range from benign cysts to malignancies of various types. Depending on the size of the mass, there may be hyperinflation or atelectasis distal to the site of obstruction. Wheezing does not respond to a bronchodilator. Treatment is of the underlying condition.

Webs and Membranes

These are congenital lesions that arise at lines of tissue fusion during embryogenesis. Webs and membranes arise from incomplete cannulization of the lumen at the junction of proximal and distal portions of airways. These structures will also cause a fixed obstruction. Often, there is no associated respiratory distress, and the signs will improve as the patient grows and airways become bigger. If there are sequelae, such as atelectasis, a surgical correction may be needed.

Laryngeal Dysfunction

Vocal cord dysfunction (VCD) is a condition in which there is closure of the vocal cords on exhalation. Normally, the vocal cords are widely adducted during exhalation. This conversion reaction can easily be confused with asthma. Patients may appear in severe distress, and poor air exchange will be noted on pulmonary examination. Auscultating the chest while the patient coughs will help, as posttussive prolongation of exhalation will be absent in VCD, but present in asthma. Auscultation over the trachea may make it clear that the obstruction is in the upper airway. A striking finding is of normal arterial blood gases in a patient in apparent severe distress. Pulmonary function flow-volume loop (see Chap. 11—Practical Pulmonary Function Studies) demonstrates flattening at the end of expiration and the beginning of inspiration, as seen in Figure 6-6. A more definitive diagnosis can be made by performing laryngoscopy while symptoms are present, where adduction of the vocal cords is seen during exhalation. The diagnosis is often complicated because patients with VCD often also have asthma that may be severe. Making the distinction is important. In a large series reported from National Jewish Hospital in Denver, nearly 10% of patients with VCD had apparently unwarranted endotracheal intubation for the condition.

Treatment of the condition consists of speech therapy and breathing exercises designed to relax the vocal cords and the throat area.

Laryngotracheomalacia and Bronchomalacia

This is a condition in which tracheal and bronchial cartilage is too soft to maintain patency of the

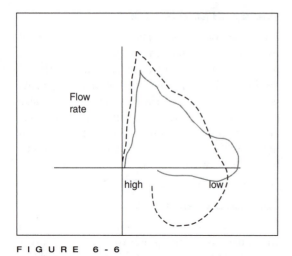

Flow rate

high   low

FLOW-VOLUME LOOP OF A PATIENT WITH VOCAL CORD DYSFUNCTION.

The normal is shown in the dashed line. Note the delay in exhalation at the end of expiration with a sudden fall in flow rate and evidence of flattening on inspiration (bottom of the graph).

airway. It is a benign condition that is seen in young infants, usually following premature birth. Endotracheal intubation may also have been needed. Inspiratory and expiratory wheezes are present. The level of clinical significance depends on how distally the airways are involved. With only the tracheal area affected, there is noisy respiration, but no clinical distress. If bronchi are involved, however, the infant may have significant collapse of the airways on exhalation, with air trapping and CO_2 retention. The work of breathing may be very high in these children, and assisted ventilation may be needed. There is usually a need for high end expiratory pressures, either as continuous positive airway pressure or as positive end expiratory pressure. A definitive diagnosis can be made on bronchoscopy, where collapse of the bronchi is seen on exhalation.

The condition usually corrects as the child grows, and bronchial cartilage becomes firmer.

Bronchopulmonary Dysplasia (BPD)

This condition is a consequence of extremely premature birth, with severe hyaline membrane disease (HMD). HMD is the result of the absence of surfactant in the lungs of premature babies, who cannot expand alveoli and develop fluid and hyaline material in the alveoli. They rapidly develop respiratory failure and very high O_2 requirement. BPD is the result of prolonged ventilation at high pressures in the presence of high inspired O_2. The result is fibrosed lung, tissue breakdown, and airway obstruction. These infants may need major long-term interventions including tracheostomy and prolonged assisted ventilation. A newborn infant has about 20% of full alveolar capacity. New lung that develops is normal, so that these children will improve as they acquire new lung tissue. However, the airway obstructive component remains as severe asthma. Older children may demonstrate a persistent obstructive picture with a reversible component on a pulmonary function study, similar to chronic obstructive pulmonary disease in smoking adults.

Infections

Pneumonia, especially viral pneumonitis, can present with wheezing and an obstructive pattern. Typical early childhood pulmonary inflammatory viruses, such as respiratory syncytial virus (RSV), parainfluenza, and adenoviruses cause an asthma-like pattern of symptoms. This is particularly true of RSV, which can lead to years of asthma-like airway obstruction, with recovery by the age of 5–6 years. Many studies have implicated RSV in the pathogenesis of asthma, especially when accompanied by early allergen exposure.

Cardiac Disease

Increased pulmonary venous engorgement from left heart failure or mitral valve disease can mimic asthma. Patients may present with wheezing and nocturnal symptoms that are very similar to asthma. The differential must be made on clinical findings of cardiac abnormalities such as a gallop rhythm or a murmur and radiographic evidence of cardiac failure (interstitial fluid, enlarged cardiac silhouette). Cardiac catheterization may be needed. In young children, congenital cardiac abnormalities often present as asthma.

Cystic Fibrosis

Cystic fibrosis is an autosomal condition that affects multiple organs, especially lungs, liver, gut, and pancreas. The gene for the condition has been identified, and a wide pattern of deletions has been delineated. The common pathway is improper water transport from the apical goblet cells which results in thickened secretions. Pulmonary involvement may resemble asthma. Persistent wheezing under the age of 6 months is particularly suspicious of cystic fibrosis. X ray may show hyperinflation and patchy infiltrates. Recurrent pneumonia is a feature of cystic fibrosis and is not seen in asthma. A frequent radiographic finding is volume loss with streaking in the upper lobes. Gastrointestinal signs are early presenting features and include meconium ileus in the newborn and intestinal obstruction. In older children, there is loss of pancreatic enzymes leading to steatorrhea with foul smelling greasy stools because of fat malabsorption.

Pilocarpine iontophoresis (*sweat test*) is the standard diagnostic test for cystic fibrosis. In children the test is positive if sweat chloride is >60 mmol/L or >80 mmol/L in adults. Ideally, two separate tests should be performed on consecutive days.

Specific DNA testing will confirm the diagnosis. This is important information for families who may consider having more children.

Other findings include the following:

- Pulmonary function studies that demonstrate decreased TLC with decreased forced vital capacity (in asthma, TLC is increased). Pulmonary diffusing capacity is normal in asthma, but reduced in cystic fibrosis.
- Fecal fat excretion is increased and serum albumin level is low.

Recurrent Aspiration

This is a problem among patients with impaired consciousness and inability to control swallow. Otherwise healthy and mentally intact people do not commonly have chronic aspiration. Repeated aspiration should be considered where the patient is retarded mentally, has neurological deficits that affect swallowing, as having a stroke, is elderly or has a history of alcohol or drug abuse. A chest radiogram may show the changes of chronic infiltration.

Confounding Variables. Asthma may be aggravated by comorbid factors and events. Examples include the following:

- Rhinitis/sinusitis
- Gastroesophageal reflux
- Aspirin sensitivity
- Sulfite sensitivity
- Beta-blockers

ASTHMA MORTALITY

Deaths from Asthma in Children

There has been an increase in the mortality rate in asthma. This change is most prominent among children living in poverty and African Americans, where the mortality rate is three times that of Whites. These data are illustrated in Figure 6-7, presented for the Midwest states of the United States. These data are representative of the country as a whole.

Potential Reasons for Recent Increase in Mortality

- General increase in severity of asthma
- Medication
  - Overuse
  - Potent combinations
  - Inadequate pharmacotherapy
  - Underuse of medications
  - Confusion due to "polypharmacy"
- Socioeconomic factors
  - Delay in seeking help
  - Cost of medication and care
  - Under-assessment of the severity of the attack
  - Decreased access to patient care

Specific Causes

- Sudden severe bronchospasm
- Spontaneous pneumothorax
- Hypoxic seizures and aspiration
- Medication toxicity
- Sudden cardiac death (rare)
  - Tamponade with hyperinflation
  - Hypokalemia

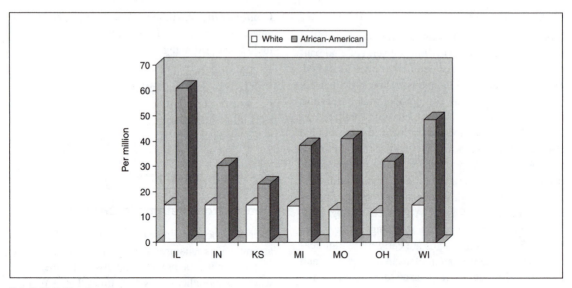

FIGURE 6-7

REPRESENTATIVE DATA FOR THE MIDWEST COMPARING MORTALITY IN ASTHMA FOR WHITES AND AFRICAN AMERICANS.

Mortality in African Americans is three times that of Whites. Midwest states are presented on the x axis using the standard abbreviations.

Source: Morbidity and Mortality Weekly Report.

ASTHMA TREATMENT

A broad approach to the management of asthma is presented here. Details of medication use and delivery are to be found in Chap. 14 on Medications and Therapeutic Methods.

Goals

Ideally, the goal of therapy is to normalize the patients' lifestyle. They should not loose sleep because of cough or wheeze, should not lose days of work or school, should not use a bronchodilator more than twice per week, should participate in sports and other activities, and should not require emergency department visits or hospitalizations.

Overall Approach

Therapy for asthma has been clearly delineated in the NAEPP. The *key aspect* of therapy is the recognition of two groups of medications with distinct uses. These are

- Reliever medications
- Controller medications

The terms refer to two key aspects of the pathophysiology, bronchospasm (early phase) and peribronchial inflammation (late phase).

Reliever Medications

This group is effective in relieving acute bronchoconstriction and is thus effective only in treating acute asthmatic episodes. There is no effect in preventing acute attacks or in preventing the effects of prolonged inflammation. These medications should only be used as needed for acute symptoms. The continuous use of albuterol or equivalent does not add to control and may be harmful.

Reliever medications fall into two groups

Beta-2 agonists
Anticholinergics

Controller Medications

This group of medications reduces the level of peribronchial inflammation and thus provides for long-term control of asthma with a reduction in the frequency of acute episodes. There are several groups of medications that fall under the heading of controllers. For details, see Chapter 16.

Steroids

- Inhaled
  - Long acting, potent inhaled steroids have made a dramatic difference in the outcome in asthma. They are intended for daily use, irrespective of the presence of symptoms.
  - Examples include
    - fluticasone (Flovent)
    - budesonide (Pulmicort)
    - beciomethasone-microfined (QVAR)
- Oral
  - In general, oral corticosteroids are reserved for acute asthmatic episodes. Long-term use should be avoided because of the high side effect profile associated with these medications.

Leukotriene modifiers

Useful as adjuncts to steroids

Can control mild to moderate asthma

Control about two-thirds of asthmatics, who presumably have a predominantly leukotriene mediated response

Mast cell stabilizing drugs. Cromolyn and Nedocromil. These drugs are weak in their effect, and are used much less often.

Methylxanthines. Once a mainstay of asthma therapy, this group of drugs has fallen into disfavor. They have a high side effect profile and are often poorly tolerated. Moreover, they are weak bronchodilators and anti-inflammatory agents.

General Approach to Therapy

The NAEPP suggest two approaches to asthma management: *step-up* and *step-down*. The level of medication is determined by the severity classification. There is controversy over when this staging should be done, and how to incorporate the influence of therapy on the classification. A constant criterion remains whether the patient has intermittent or persistent symptoms. The presence of persistent or intermittent symptoms relies on medication use and frequency of severe attacks. Based on the NAEPP, the patient with *intermittent* asthma should have the following:

- No more than two uses of a reliever medication per week
- No more than two nocturnal episodes in a month
- No more than two acute episodes in a year that require steroids orally or two emergency visits
- Not use more than one canister of a reliever medication per year

Any patient who has persistent symptoms by these criteria should be placed on a controller medication. The number and dose of medications should be such that the patient meets control criteria noted above. The suggested order of adding medications noted in the NAEPP is in Table 6-9. This is a suggested approach, and each patient should be judged on the severity of the disease, individual responses to different classes of medications and the level of clinical and pulmonary function control.

Step-Up

In this approach, the patient's regimen becomes increasingly complex with added medications to maintain control.

Step-Down

The patient is placed on an aggressive regimen to control the disease, and the medications are then

TABLE 6-9

THIS IS A PRESENTATION OF TYPICAL REGIMENS FOR TREATING VARIOUS LEVELS OF ASTHMA SEVERITY AS SUGGESTED BY THE NAEPP

Mild intermittent	prn beta agonist
Mild to moderate persistent	Inhaled anti-inflammatory agent
	Long acting beta agonist
	Theophylline
Severe persistent	Above plus
	High dose inhaled anti-inflammatory drug
	Oral corticosteroids

"stepped down" to the least amount needed to maintain control (Table 6-9).

Acute Management at Home

Figure 6-4 presents an approach to acute asthma (after NAEPP) for rapid initiation of home therapy.

One of the major advances in the management of asthma is the inception of early management at home. It is clear that the earlier that the patient treats an acute episode of asthma, the better the outcome will be. The patient should be encouraged to use rescue medication even if they are unsure that it is needed.

The algorithm adapted from NAEPP in Figure 6-4 is intended as a guide only, and each acute episode may need an individualized approach. If there is any doubt in the patient's or parent's mind about the appropriate mode of therapy, they should contact a physician or call for an ambulance. Patients having acute respiratory distress *should never be transported to an emergency department by private car.*

The patient's initial response to an acute episode is to use an inhalation treatment either by metered dose inhaler (MDI) or by nebulizer, as fits the patient's ability to use an MDI when having respiratory difficulties. If there is a good response, then the patient should continue using albuterol every 4–6 hours for 48 hours and reassess. The physician should be notified.

In the case of a partial response, the patient should start an oral corticosteroid, and repeat the inhaled bronchodilator three times in the first hour. If there is still only a partial response, the patient should be seen in the emergency department or by their physician. If the patient responds, they should continue with the bronchodilator for 2–3 days, and discuss the acute episode with their physician. If the patient shows a poor or no response to inhaled bronchodilator therapy in the first hour, they should start oral corticosteroid therapy. This patient must be seen immediately in the emergency department or by the primary care doctor and should take inhaled beta-2 agonist therapy continuously (Table 6-10).

TABLE 6-10

ASSESSMENT OF AN ACUTE ASTHMATIC EPISODE FOR LEVEL OF SEVERITY

	Mild	Moderate	Severe	Impending Failure
Breathless	Walking	Talking feeding	Rest	
	Can lie down	Sitting	Hunched	
Talks in	Sentences	Phrases	Words	
Alert	Yes	Agitated	Agitated+	Drowsy confused
Respiration	+	+ +	+ + +	
Heart rate	+	+ +	+ + +	
Accessory muscles	±	+	+ +	Paradoxical
Air exchange	Good	Reduced on expiration	Reduced+	Very poor
Wheeze	Mild	Loud	Louder	Absent
Pulsus paradoxus	<10 torr	10–20 torr	>20 torr	May be absent
Peak flow	>80%	50–80%	<50%	
SaO$_2$	>95%	91–95%	<90%	
PaCO$_2$	<45 torr	<45 torr	<60 torr	>60 torr
PaO$_2$	Normal	>60 torr	<60 torr	

Source: Adapted from International Consensus Report.
Note: This table is intended to supplement an assessment by the physician.

Table 6-10 is a summation of the assessment of the patient having an acute asthmatic episode presenting in the emergency department or physician's office. This is a guide, and should not replace the physician's assessment of the level of illness of the patient.

Therapy—Medications

Delivery Systems

(For further details, see Therapy chapter.)

There are three routes of administration of asthma medications: oral, inhaled, and parenteral.

The inhaled route is the most used. Unfortunately, a profusion of devices and mechanisms has emerged for the delivery of medication by this route, resulting in confusion about their use.

Inhalation devices. There are three main groups of delivery systems:

- Metered dose inhaler (MDI)
- Dry powder inhaler (DPI)
- Nebulizer

Action Plan. The NAEPP recommends the use of an action plan. This plan is based on the peak flow and uses the inverted traffic light values noted above. The green, yellow and red zones are based on the patient's best peak flow, since many patients may never reach predicted values (see Table 6-7).

CLINICAL SCENARIOS

The following cases illustrate an approach to managing patients with different severity and presentation of asthma.

Case 1

This is a case of a 4-year-old girl who presents with a history of recurrent pneumonia. These episodes are characterized by:

- Upper respiratory tract infections
- Harsh, barking cough at night, even when she does not have an infection. Cough occurs three to four times per week
- Cough with activity, tires easily when playing with friends

- Scattered crackles on pulmonary examination, prolonged exhalation
- Patchy infiltrates by chest x ray, hyperinflation
- Normal CBC with acute episodes, no bandemia

Explanation

This child has asthma with a predominant cough expression. Her episodes are triggered by upper respiratory infections and activity. The clues are the recurrent nature of the pulmonary episodes and the frequent nocturnal symptoms. Recurrent pneumonia is an unusual event in children, and one should first suspect another etiology for the respiratory symptoms. The infiltrates are probably subsegmental atelectasis as part of asthma.

Management

- Trial of therapy with albuterol. This should be given for 1 week, and resolution of symptoms noted. Improvement of cough with albuterol is an indicator of reversible symptoms, a criterion of asthma.
- Controller medications.
  - Pulmicort Respules 250 μg bid if the patient has persistent symptoms, increase to 500 μg bid and reduce once symptoms are controlled.
  - Singulair 4 mg daily.
  - Albuterol as needed.
  - Oral steroids may be needed for refractory acute episodes of cough or "pneumonia."
- Investigation.
  - Subsequent chest x ray should only be obtained if there is a specific question to answer.
  - Allergy testing should be considered. It is useful to delineate the response pattern and allergens that can be avoided. The presence of positive allergy tests and a family history increases the likelihood that the asthma symptoms will persist beyond 6 years of age.
  - Allergen avoidance, environmental controls.
- Reducing medication.
  - Once the patient has not had symptoms for 4–6 months, medication can be reduced. If she remains symptom free, she can attempt to discontinue Pulmicort. If there is a seasonal

pattern, she can use Pulmicort during the season, if that is when she has symptoms.

- Pulmicort daily.
- Continue singulair.

Case 2

A 22-year-old male college student is very athletic, but has recently developed difficulty with distance events. He now cannot complete a mile run, whereas he previously held the state record for this event.

He has been advised to use two inhalations of albuterol which he takes by closed mouth technique immediately prior to exercise, but is still not competing at optimal level. He is at risk for being dropped from the team.

Pulmonary function studies (see Chap. 11) indicate normal baseline values. With an exercise challenge test performed on a treadmill, FEV1 was reduced by 30% after only 4 minutes of low intensity activity. Following inhalation of albuterol, FEV1 returns to within 90% of predicted normal. This is a strongly positive exercise challenge

Explanation

What is implied by the lack of response to albuterol? Exercise triggered asthma is not a separate form of asthma. This young man has uncontrolled asthma, but his trigger is mainly exercise. It is also likely that his technique for using albuterol is poor, and he is not receiving an adequate dose.

Management

This patient will benefit from a step-down approach to therapy. The idea is to gain control of his symptoms, and then decrease medication to the least amount needed. He should start on Advair 250/50–500/50 μg bid and Singulair 10 mg daily. If he has symptoms during sports or other activities, he should use albuterol for rescue. Maxair Autohaler would be a good alternative if his technique is poor with albuterol.

A useful adjunct would be for him to use a peak flow meter. He should establish a baseline peak flow, and use it as an objective guide when he has difficulty while exercising. He should follow the standard action plan response to the peak flow zones.

As his symptoms improve, he can reduce the medication to Advair 100/50 μg. He can then transition to Flovent or Pulmicort Turbuhaler and use Serevent on days when he exercises.

Case 3

A 14-year-old AA female with severe asthma has had numerous hospitalizations, a total of 17 to the Intensive Care Unit. She has required endotracheal intubation and assisted ventilation three times. She developed spontaneous pneumothorax. She has monthly clinic visits and appears to be compliant with medication.

Therapy consists of daily oral steroids, occasionally every other day, inhaled beclomethasone 348 μg tid oral theophylline and salmeterol bid. She lives in an area with a high antigen and pollution load. There are no animals or smokers in the house.

She had comorbid factors: sinusitis and gastroesophageal reflux.

Explanation

- Why is she refractory to therapy? While the reasons for patients being steroid resistant are not clear, this patient has several problems.
- She falls into a high risk category based on race and age.
- She lives in conditions that result in a high level of exposure to pollution and allergens.
- She has sinusitis and gastroesophageal reflux which increase morbidity in asthma. Reflux in particular increases bronchial tone and causes narrowed airways.

Management

The underlying sinus disease should be treated, as should the reflux. Medical management is a first option. The extent of sinus disease can be determined by a CT scan and the appropriate therapy instituted. Reflux should be managed initially with a proton pump inhibitor such as omeprazole (Prilosec). Surgical correction can be considered if there is no response, but asthma is often not helped by antireflux surgery.

Advair would be a good choice (500/50 μg) because there seems to be an advantage to the combination and it is easier to take than the components separately. Beclomethasone should be stopped. Singulair 10 mg should be added. She could continue theophylline, as there are data that indicate that this drug may have a steroid sparing effect at low concentrations.

The patient could be maintained on every other day steroids, which may be easier to achieve with fluticasone than beclomethasone.

This group of patients remain very difficult to manage, and are at high risk. The importance of taking medication and regular follow-up must be emphasized repeatedly.

Case 4

This is a 40-year-old woman who has apparently been in good health. She exercises moderately and does not smoke cigarettes. She has noticed sneezing, itchy eyes, and mild respiratory distress when around cats. She also has problems with weather changes and has noticed that the tightness occurs when she goes from a heated environment into cold air. She continues to exercise without difficulty.

Physical examination reveals allergic shiners, pale blue nasal mucosa and a cobblestone appearance to the pharynx. Pulmonary examination is generally normal, and the remainder of the physical examination is normal.

Pulmonary function testing indicates a mild reduction in FEV1 to 75% and there is a 12% change with a bronchodilator.

Allergy testing indicates positive reactions to cat and dog dander, house dust mites, and several molds. She also reacts to tree and grass pollen.

Explanation

- This patient has allergic rhinitis with asthma. Her asthma appears mild to moderate.
- Therapy should include
  - Avoidance measures. If this is not possible, selected allergy immunotherapy to cats is an option since there is a clear history of reactions on exposure.
  - Environmental control, including bedding protection and filtering air from the furnace and air conditioner.

- It is reasonable to use a step-up approach initially in this patient, starting with a leukotriene modifier. This should show an effect within 1–2 weeks. If there is no response, or a minimal response, an inhaled steroid should be added. Once the patient is controlled, medication can again be stepped down.
- A topical nasal steroid, such as fluticasone, beclomethasone, or mometasone should be used. A second generation antihistamine like desloratadine, cetirizine, or fexofenadine should be used for symptoms.
- Frequent follow-up is indicated. Pulmonary function is essential in following this patient.

Suggested Reading

Bradding, P. (2003). The role of the mast cell in asthma: a reassessment. *Curr Opin Allergy Clin Immunol* **3**(1): 45–50.

Ennis, M. (2003). Neutrophils in asthma pathophysiology. *Curr Allergy Asthma Rep* **3**(2): 159–65.

Factor, P. (2003). Gene therapy for asthma. *Mol Ther* **7**(2): 148–52.

Fireman, P. (2003). Understanding asthma pathophysiology. *Allergy Asthma Proc* **24**(2): 79–83.

Flaherty, K. R., E. A. Kazerooni, et al. (2000). Differential diagnosis of chronic airflow obstruction. *J Asthma* **37**(3): 201–23.

Hizawa, N., L. R. Freidhoff, Y. E. Chiu et al. (1998). Genetic regulation of dermatophagoides pteronyssinus-specific IgE responsiveness: a genome-wide multipoint linkage analysis in families recruited through 2 asthmatic sibs. *J Allergy Clin Immunol* **102**(3): 436–42.

Hizawa N., I. R. Freidhoff, E. Ehrlich et al. (1998). Genetic influences of chromosomes 5q31-q33 and 11q13 on specific IgE responsiveness to common inhaled allergens among African American families. *J Allergy Clin Immunol* **102**(3): 449–53.

King, T. E., Jr. (1999). A new look at the pathophysiology of asthma. *J Natl Med Assoc* **91**(8 Suppl.): 9S–15S.

Quadrelli, S. A., A. J. Roncoroni, et al. (1999). Evaluation of bronchodilator response in patients with airway obstruction. *Respir Med* **93**(9): 630–6.

Steinke, J. W., L. Borish, et al. (2003). 5. Genetics of hypersensitivity[erratum appears in J Allergy Clin Immunol. 2003 Aug;112(2):267]. *J Allergy Clin Immunol* **111**(2 Suppl.): S495–501.

Wenzel, S. (2003). Severe asthma: epidemiology, pathophysiology and treatment. *Mt Sinai J Med* **70**(3): 185–90.

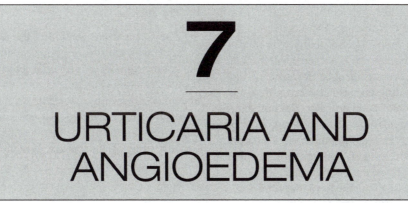

7

URTICARIA AND ANGIOEDEMA

INTRODUCTION

Urticaria and angioedema are common forms of allergic swelling. By some estimates, they involve more than 25% of the general population. Most of the time, the episodes are self-limited. Acute episodes are more common in children, while chronic forms occur more in adults. The cause is often difficult to determine, and detection depends on a careful history. This can be a very frustrating condition for the physician and patient, especially in recurrent form. The response to therapy is variable, increasing the management difficulties.

PATHOPHYSIOLOGY

Urticaria and angioedema are dependent on the same allergic mechanism. This response is mediated by IgE and depends on prior sensitization. These molecules of IgE are fixed to mast cells in a random distribution throughout the body. There is a higher concentration on skin, gut, and pulmonary mast cells. An antigen can gain access to circulation by absorption from gastrointestinal tract, skin, respiratory tract, or site of injection or insect sting. Ingested proteins can pass intact into the germinal centers in small bowel via thin-walled M cells

overlying these Peyer's patches. There are no microvilli in the region of germinal centers.

The antigen binds specifically to IgE on mast cells, causing cross-linking of the IgE molecules. This causes distortion of the membrane, which results in activation of phosphorylcholine and other enzymes in the membrane. The result is the opening of calcium channels and the controlled disintegration of the mast cell, releasing histamine and eosinophil chemoattractant molecules. This is a very rapid process that occurs within milliseconds of binding of antigen. Since they are synthesized de novo, the leukotrienes and prostaglandins take relatively longer to exert an effect than does histamine. (As a group, the leukotrienes and prostaglandins were previously known as the Slow-Reacting Substance of Anaphylaxis).

There are alternative mechanisms for mast cell degranulation. Many substances cause degranulation by a direct effect on the membrane. Examples are strawberries, iodine containing contrast media, and opiates. Conditions that cause breakdown of the complement pathway release byproducts, such as C3a and C5a which bind to specific receptors on mast cells and basophils and cause rapid release of vasoactive mediators. These complement components are potent anaphylotoxins and can induce profound shock. Complement activation occurs in diseases where soluble immune complexes are found in circulation. Examples are serum sickness and systemic lupus erythematosus.

The result of this release of vasoactive mediators is increased vascular permeability with transudation of fluid which leads to local edema and swelling. The process is identical for urticaria and angioedema; the difference is in the layer of skin in which the fluid collects. In urticaria, fluid accumulates within the epidermis. This leads to tearing of the tissue plane, and development of a sharply defined wheal. Because of the stimulation of fine sensory nerve endings, these lesions induce intense pruritus. In the case of angioedema, the fluid accumulates at the dermoepidermal junction. This is a natural cleavage plane, so that the fluid is not confined and can track widely. The clinical result is diffuse swelling which usually occurs in sites of loose connective tissue such as lips, face, tongue, extremities, and pudendal area. If the swelling occurs in the larynx, respiration may be compromised. Larger sensory nerves are stimulated in angioedema because the fluid is deeper in the skin, giving rise to a painful or burning sensation.

Anaphylaxis represents an extreme of this response. Binding of antigen to a high density of specific IgE on mast cells results in the sudden release of a large quantity of vasoactive mediators. This reaction causes vasodilation and shock, potentially within minutes.

CLINICAL FINDINGS

Patients characteristically present with sudden onset of swelling or hives. The lesions can begin at any site, not necessarily related to the poral of entry. The spread and distribution of the lesions depends on the prior attachment of IgE to mast cells. There are three important features that suggest an IgE mediated reaction:

- Rapid onset of symptoms, usually within 30 minutes.
- Apparent dose independence; a small dose can cause as strong a reaction as a large dose. This phenomenon is because the dilution curve is

shifted into the nanogram range, and the titration curve is flat at clinical doses.
- Pruritus.

The size and distribution of the lesions do not correlate with the severity or cause of the reaction, nor do the number of urticarial lesions. Urticarial lesions are evanescent, raised, sharply demarcated, and intensely pruritic. Patients with angioedema may have rapid swelling that can cause compromised function or be life threatening. This is particularly true of the larynx, mouth and tongue, where rapid swelling will cause airway obstruction.

History

Essential Features in the History

A careful history is essential in investigating urticaria.

Onset of the Reaction

The patient or parent should be asked about possible precipitating agents, such as food or medications. Since most IgE mediated reactions occur within 30 minutes of exposure, concentrating on that period is useful, and is easier for the patient to remember exposures. Patients are often asked what new exposures they might have had. This line of questioning is not helpful, as an IgE mediated reaction requires prior sensitization and thus an initial exposure will not cause a reaction. As a corollary, a reaction to a new food or other substance is probably the result of another mechanism.

Events Surrounding the Onset

Asking about difficulty talking or swallowing or breathing will give an indication of the severity of the reaction and whether the patient is at risk for a life-threatening episode.

If the patient has had multiple episodes, it is useful to determine the usual course.

One should inquire whether the patient has required emergency department care, and what medication was given. The use of steroids in the past implies a more severe episode.

The response to medication and the duration of symptoms are useful in assessing the severity.

Patients who have recurrent episodes should be encouraged to keep a diary and note foods and other possible triggers with the episodes. Urticaria is regarded as chronic when episodes persist for longer than 6 weeks.

Patients may present with

Swelling of the face, lips, tongue
Laryngeal edema
Swelling at other body sites
Urticaria sharply demarcated, pruritic
Angioedema diffuse swelling, painful

Causes

Most urticarial reactions are caused by food or medication. Reactions to food can result from a variety of antigens, some of which may be destroyed by heat and cooking. Patients may thus note that they react to an uncooked or partly cooked food, but not when it is thoroughly cooked. Foods may be cooked in the same oil or on the same grill, such as fish and hamburgers. An unsuspecting patient who is fish allergic may have a severe reaction when eating a hamburger that may contain only minute traces of fish protein. Typical foods that cause reactions are dairy products, especially milk and eggs, shellfish, peanuts and nuts, and berries. Some foods, like tomatoes, contain serotonin and other histamine-like agents. There are also other poorly identified substances that trigger mast cell degranulation and can cause direct histamine-like effects (Table 7-1).

Foods

Dairy products. Cow's milk and related milk products are very frequently identified as a cause of allergies. The exact frequency is difficult to ascertain, because other causes of similar symptoms, such as lactose deficiency, are confused with IgE mediated reactions. In infants, there are often two types of milk allergic reactions. Local milk reactions in the gut cause cramping, diarrhea, and emesis. The symptoms occur soon after milk ingestion, and the diarrhea is often bloody. In infants who have high anti cow's milk IgE, there are often upper airway symptoms with persistent rhinorrhea and sometimes wheezing (see also the chapter on Food Allergy).

TABLE 7.1

COMMON CAUSES OF URTICARIA AND ANGIOEDEMA

Foods
Dairy products
Peanuts
Nuts and berries
Seafood
Drugs
IgE mediated
Penicillin
Sulfa drugs
Direct release of histamine
Opiates
Iodides
Physical
Stress
Solar
Vibration
Cold
Hereditary
C1 esterase inhibitor deficiency
C3b inhibitor deficiency

Eggs are also common as causes of urticaria and angioedema. There is a further problem with eggs, in that many vaccines are developed in eggs. Examples are measles, mumps and rubella, and influenza vaccines. These vaccines must be given with caution in egg allergic patients.

Peanuts. Peanuts are actually legumes, and are distinct from tree nuts. They contain several potent allergens, that may be enhanced by roasting. Peanuts are a major cause of marked allergic reactions, including anaphylaxis. Patients who have a high level of antipeanut IgE can develop shock within seconds of the slightest contact with a peanut.

Nuts and berries. All tree nuts (almonds, hazelnuts, cashews, pecans, and walnuts, for example) can cause serious reactions. Many seeds that are commonly used in food, especially sesame seeds, often cause severe reactions. There is cross-reactivity among nuts and seeds in the same families. However, not all reactions are predictable. Peanuts and sesame seeds can cross-react and peanut allergic patients should be cautious with seeds and nuts.

Many berries cause reactions. Some, such as strawberries cause direct release of histamine and are not mediated via IgE.

Seafood and fish. Seafood includes shrimp, crab, lobster, and bivalves including oysters and clams. Reactions to shrimp occur in an IgE mediated form, which is to proteins such as tropomyosin. There is cross-reactivity with other arthropods, such as mite and cockroaches. There are people who can eat shelled shrimp, but react if they handle the shells.

Reactions to crustacea, including crab and lobster, are separate from shrimp. Patients may react to one and not the other.

Reactions to fish are usually common across different species. If a person reacts to one type of fish, they will often react to many, and should be advised to avoid fish completely.

Drugs. Reactions to medications fall into two groups:

IgE mediated

Penicillin: Reactions to penicillins are very common. There are two types. Reactions occur to the central beta lactam ring, known as the *major determinant*, and to various breakdown products which form the *minor determinants*. In general, severe responses occur with parenteral route of administration. There is strong cross-reactivity among beta lactam ring antibiotics, such as cephalosporins and carbapenems. Penicillins are the most frequent medication that causes anaphylaxis.

Sulfa drugs: Reactions to sulfa containing compounds are common and usually present as urticaria and angioedema. Sulfonamides may not cross-react with other sulfa drugs.

Direct release of histamine

Opiates: Opiates are a prime example of agents that directly cause mast cells to disintegrate. The degree of reaction is an idiosyncrasy, and is not related to prior sensitization. Almost all patients will have pruritus following administration of opiates, especially morphine.

Radiocontrast: The reaction to hypertonic iodine containing radiocontrast materials is a direct effect on mast cells, although the exact mechanism has not been elucidated. The reaction is difficult to predict, but a test dose of the contrast material should be given before injection. There is no reliable in vitro diagnostic test for this reaction.

Salicylate: Angioedema occurs in sensitive individuals who use salicylates. The lesions are not pruritic and often involve the face and eyelids. Sampter's triad consists of sinusitis, angioedema, and asthma and probably results from an imbalance in the production of prostaglandins, perhaps with increased leukotriene synthesis.

Physical

Dermographism. This is a nonpathologic disorder. A wheal and flare response can be induced by light stroking of the skin. Patients often develop urticarial lesions from contact with clothing. This is a benign condition that is usually self-limited and is not associated with severe reactions.

Stress. Emotional and physical stress can both trigger acute urticarial reactions in susceptible individuals. The mechanism probably relates to autonomic imbalances that accompany stress.

Cholinergic. The urticaria of cholinergic syndromes is typical. There is a cluster of punctate wheals surrounded by a flare response. Sometimes, a central wheal with satellite lesions is seen. As a diagnostic test, methacholone can be injected intradermally. In a positive result, the typical pattern of a wheal with satellite lesions will be reproduced.

Cold. There are several forms of cold urticaria, including a familial variety and several that are associated with cryoglobulins and other cold reacting serum proteins. Patients have problems when exposed on cold days, to cold water, and to sudden changes in temperature. They have typical cholinergic urticaria, and in severe cases can develop shock. Anaphylaxis is more likely in total immersion, as in swimming. They present with a cholinergic type pattern of urticarial lesions.

Heat. Exposure to heat sources, such as hot shower, can cause a cholinergic urticarial reaction in predisposed individuals.

Solar. In sensitive individuals, exposure to light in the infrared range can induce cholinergic type urticaria.

Vibration. Workers exposed to heavy, repeated vibration, as in the use of jackhammers, may develop urticaria of exposed areas. A pattern of urticaria involving the hands and forearms of a construction worker is suggestive of this type of repeated trauma.

Unusual disorders

Mastocytosis. There are several categories of mastocytosis which present in very similar ways. Skin, GI tract, lymph nodes, liver, spleen, and bone marrow are the most frequent source of problems. In this disorder, there is a marked increase in the density of mast cells in the skin and other organs. Most urticarial or angioedema episodes occur spontaneously but reactions, including anaphylaxis may be provoked by any triggers of mast cell degranulation such as alcohol, aspirin, insect stings, infection, or exposure to iodinated contrast materials.

Urticaria Pigmentosa: This is the most common skin manifestation of mastocytosis. The lesions appear on the trunk and limbs as small yellowish-tan to reddish-brown macules or slightly raised papules. In young children, the lesions may be bullous. The palms, soles, face, and scalp are spared. *Darier's sign* is elicited by rubbing the lesions with resulting urticaria. GI tract symptoms occur commonly (50–80%), with abdominal pain and diarrhea.

Hereditary

C1 esterase inhibitor deficiency
C3b inhibitor deficiency

Hereditary angioedema. This is an uncommon disorder that is due to a defect in the serum protease inhibitor, *C1 esterase inhibitor*. This enzyme prevents the activation of the first complement component, C1, by the cleaving enzyme, C1 esterase. The condition is inherited as an autosomal dominant condition.

Symptoms are generally triggered by exposure to cold or by trauma. The sites that are involved are lips, tongue, face, hands, and feet. There is prominent angioedema, with marked lip swelling. Urticaria does not occur in this condition. Patients may experience laryngeal edema and acute respiratory distress which can be life threatening. Gut mucosa is often involved, with edema and swelling causing acute abdominal pain and cramping.

The mechanism whereby activation of C1 esterase results in edema is not clear. Components of the complement cascade such as C3a and C5a are potent at causing mast cells to degranulate. It is not clear in vivo, however, that this is the mechanism.

Types

Genetic: There are two genetic forms of the condition:

Type I: Eighty-five percent of all patients. In this form of the disease, production and function of the C1 esterase inhibitor protein is markedly reduced, to levels of 5–50 percent of normal.

Type II: In this form of the condition there are normal levels of C1 inhibitor but functional activity is markedly reduced.

Acquired: Acquired hereditary angioedema results from complement depletion in diseases where there is formation of soluble immune complexes, as in lupus erythematosus or lymphoproliferative disorders.

Clinical presentation. Patients present with abrupt onset of angioedema. Swelling generally progresses over 24–48 hours, and then regresses slowly.

Involved areas are usually the following:

- Around the face, lips, and hands.
- The pharynx and oropharynx may be involved, and laryngeal edema is a significant risk.
- Gastrointestinal involvement results in abdominal pain, cramping, and diarrhea. This presentation may be mistaken for an acute abdomen.

Other features

- Fever and leukocytosis are generally absent.
- Swelling episodes are usually triggered by exposure to cold or by minor trauma.
- Fifty percent of patients are usually symptomatic by early adolescence.

Therapy

- Initial therapy with epinephrine, especially in high risk reactions such as laryngeal edema, can be life saving. In general, however, there is not a good response to adrenergic agents.
- Antihistamines and corticosteroids are ineffective in treating this condition.
- Androgenic steroids such as danazol stimulate synthesis of C1 inhibitor. Dosage should be titrated to the minimum level required. The use of these drugs is particularly problematic in early teenage girls. Their use is usually limited to patients who have severe reactions that are potentially life threatening.
- Antithrombotic agents, such as epsilon amino caproic acid have some effect in decreasing complement activation.

Chronic Urticaria

Chronic urticaria is defined as allergic swelling that continues for longer than 6 weeks.

Pathology

- Histopathology often demonstrates a vasculitic response.
- There is transudation of fluid into the perivascular space.

Causes

This condition raises concerns about the possibility of underlying pathology. This is particularly an issue because the mechanism of many of the potential causes involves the formation of circulating immune complexes. One of the side effects of immune complexes is the activation of mast cells with the release of histamine and other acute inflammatory mediators. Underlying conditions that may cause chronic urticaria are shown in Table 7-2.

TABLE 7.2

A LIST OF CONDITIONS THAT ARE ASSOCIATED WITH CHRONIC URTICARIA

Rheumatoid Diseases
Systemic lupus erythematosus
Inflammatory bowel diseases
Malignancy
Solid cancers
Lymphoid malignancies
Thyroid Disease
Hashimoto's disease particularly
Sensitivity
NSAIDs
Aspirin

Note: Over 80% of chronic urticaria remains idiopathic.

Most of the possible underlying conditions mentioned above are actually rare as causes of chronic urticaria or angioedema. Hashimoto's disease is the exception, and is the one possibility that should be investigated, especially in young women with chronic urticaria.

Delineation of etiology. The cause is generally obscure and 80% of chronic cases are classified as idiopathic. Reviews of the demographics of chronic urticaria and angioedema indicate that

- 61% are women with a mean age of 40 years
- 56% are idiopathic
- 15% are physical
- 10% are intolerant of salicylates
- 44% may responded to H1 antagonists

INVESTIGATION

Acute

History

A careful history is essential. Events within 30 minutes of onset of the rash or swelling are usually most relevant. Previous exposure without a reaction does not exclude a particular agent from consideration.

Diary. Having the patient maintain a daily food diary and noting when reactions occur can be a useful method to detect patterns when urticaria and angioedema occur. The diary is best kept in 2-week blocks, to improve compliance.

Laboratory Tests

Allergy tests

Total IgE. The total IgE does not add to the diagnosis, and is of little value.

Specific IgE

Prick skin test: The value of specific IgE in determining the etiology of urticaria and angioedema depends on the type of suspected antigen.

For suspected food antigens, allergy testing by in vitro or in vivo methods is about 90–95% predictive of a negative reaction to the food but only 65% for a positive reaction. This means that a positive test without a history of reaction to that food is not clinically significant. On the other hand, a negative test to a food that the patient or parent suspects is a strong indication that the food is not the cause of urticaria.

In general, clinical in vivo testing is preferable and is more significant than in vitro testing. In the case of urticaria and angioedema, however, the skin may have an abnormal reaction to antigens and is therefore often not suitable.

RAST: The RAST (radioallergosorbent test) or a variant (see chapter Diagnostic Methods for details) is sensitive for the detection of small quantities of specific circulating IgE. The RAST is preferable to prick skin test where the skin is extensively involved and is unreliable as a measure of specific IgE release.

When there is a history of a severe reaction to a suspected antigen and it is dangerous to place the antigen on the patient's skin, the RAST should be chosen.

Chronic

Further Investigations

In chronic urticaria, and where there is a suspicion of an underlying disease, further investigation

may be useful. It is worth noting that the yield from these investigations is very small; they are not justified in the absence of a suggestive history.

Complete blood count and differential. The presence of eosinophils indicates the possibility of the presence of allergy, drug reaction, or parasitic infestations. (The converse is also true; in the absence of eosinophils, the possibility of a parasitic infection is less of a consideration.)

Sedimentation rate and c-reactive protein (CRP). Elevation of the ESR indicates that there is a systemic process as a cause of the urticaria. An elevated CRP indicates the presence of chronic inflammation, increasing the likelihood of a systemic cause of chronic urticaria.

Tests for rheumatoid diseases

Rheumatoid factor
Antinuclear antibody test
Antidouble-stranded DNA

Stool for ova and parasites. These are uncommon causes for chronic urticaria and angioedema. This investigation should be reserved for patients who have gastrointestinal symptoms such as blood in the stool, chronic diarrhea, or malabsorption syndrome.

Skin biopsy. Skin biopsy will help detect the presence of vasculitis. A biopsy in urticaria will show edema in the perivascular space, without vascular involvement. The finding of vascular damage and inflammatory changes, such as lymphocytic and polymorphonuclear infiltrate suggests another etiology, possibly a rheumatoid condition.

THERAPY

See chapter on Therapy for details and dosing of medications.

Immediate Therapy of Urticaria and Angioedema

Antihistamines

Initial therapy should be with an antihistamine. First generation drugs such as diphenhydramine

(Benadryl) or hydroxyzine (Atarax, Vistaril) at doses from 75 to 200 mg per day. Second generation antihistamines (loratadine—Claritin, cetirizine—Zyrtec and fexofenadine—Allegra) have the advantage of not being sedating and lasting 24 hours. However, they are less effective in many instances than the first generation drugs. The sedating effect and strong anticholinergic properties of the Benadryl and Atarax are advantageous in controlling pruritus.

Epinephrine

Epinephrine may be needed acutely if there is respiratory compromise, rapidly progressive swelling, or diaphoresis. Subcutaneous or intramuscular injection of 0.01 mL/kg up to 0.3–0.5 cc of a 1/1000 (1 mg/mL) dilution should be given while other measures are instituted. The dose can be repeated twice at 20-minute intervals.

Steroids

For more severe acute symptoms, corticosteroid therapy should be instituted. A dose of prednisone, 1 mg/kg to 60 mg per day is effective, and can be continued for 3–5 days. Alternatively, methylprednisolone (Medrol) can be used in a tapering dose over 5 days in the same dose range.

Chronic Urticaria

The goal in chronic urticaria is to provide symptomatic relief until the condition resolves spontaneously.

Antihistamines

Antihistamines are effective in reducing pruritus, but may not significantly reduce the occurrence of lesions. In addition, other first generation antihistamines, such as cyproheptadine (Periactin) and Doxepin are effective in cholinergic urticaria. These drugs are particularly sedating, but gradually increasing the dose can ameliorate this side effect.

A combination of cyproheptadine (Periactin) and hydroxyzine may give greater relief than either drug alone will do. A typical regimen might be 25 mg of hydroxyzine and 4 mg of cyproheptadine taken together qid. A maximal daily dosage of 200 mg of hydroxyzine and 32 mg of cyproheptadine can be given based on the frequency and severity of outbreaks. Doxepin has its supporters because it also possesses some H_2 blocking properties. However, it is particularly sedating and might best be used as a nighttime dose of 25–50 mg as a supplement to antihistaminics. Patients can sometimes tolerate side effects of one antihistamine better than those of another, even though the doses used are comparable. Some experimentation may be needed to find the combination that works for a particular patient. Finding the right combination of antihistamines can usually ameliorate the worst symptoms of chronic urticaria; the pruritus and alarming skin lesions. The patient can be reasonably comfortable and function normally.

Non-sedating antihistamines such as desloratadine (Clarinex 5 mg) or cetirizine (Zyrtec 10 mg) are not always as effective as the more sedating compounds. However, many milder cases of urticaria may be treated with these agents. Combinations with sedating antihistamines used at night are often successful.

The addition of specific histamine H_2 receptor blockers is useful in controlling the vasodilatation component of chronic urticaria. Skin blood vessels have H_2 receptors. Cimetidine (Tagamet) 300 mg qid or ranitidine (Zantec) 150 mg twice a day are possible dosing regimens. About 3 weeks can be considered a reasonable trial of these medications.

Corticosteroids

The addition of a corticosteroid may be necessary to control urticaria. The lowest possible effective dosage should be used. Possible dosing schedules are presented in the chapter on Therapy. A daily starting dose of 1–2 mg/kg will usually control symptoms. This starting dose can be continued for 5 days, and then tapered to an alternate day dosing schedule. The alternate day dosing should be slowly tapered, monitoring the presence of lesions. Ideally, the patient should be symptom free before withdrawing the alternate day dose completely. Antihistamines should be continued with the corticosteroid and should probably not be tapered until the patient no longer requires the steroid. In cases where the patient has lesions on the day of not taking steroids, dividing the dose on the day of scheduled steroids will be helpful. An example is 30 mg prednisone in the morning and 10 mg in the evening. Using a steroid without mineralocorticoid effects, as with methylprednisolone, can reduce the side effects.

Anabolic Steroids

The use of a semisynthetic anabolic steroid, danazol, is helpful in hereditary angioedema. Its use presents dilemmas in teenage girls with the disease, and it should be reserved for patients who have life-threatening episodes.

Specific Therapy

Where an underlying disease is present, therapy should be directed at the cause. In this case, treatment of chronic urticaria is adjunctive to therapy of the cause of the lesions, for example, systemic lupus erythematosus.

Suggested Reading

Black, A. K. and M. W. Greaves (2002). Antihistamines in urticaria and angioedema. *Clin Allergy Immunol* **17**: 249–86.

Burks, W. (2003). Skin manifestations of food allergy. *Pediatrics* **111**(6 Pt. 3): 1617–24.

Charlesworth, E. N. (2002). Urticaria and angioedema. *Allergy Asthma Proc* **23**(5): 341–5.

Condemi, J. J. (2002). Allergic reactions to natural rubber latex at home, to rubber products, and to cross-reacting foods. *J Allergy Clin Immunol* **110** (2 Suppl.): S107–10.

Greaves, M. W. (2002). Pathophysiology of chronic urticaria. *Int Arch Allergy Immunol* **127**(1): 3–9.

Kagi, M. K. (2001). Leukotriene receptor antagonists—a novel therapeutic approach in atopic dermatitis? *Dermatology* **203**(4): 280–3.

Roelandts, R. (2003). Diagnosis and treatment of solar urticaria. *Dermatol Ther* **16**(1): 52–6.

Rottem, M. (2003). Chronic urticaria and autoimmune thyroid disease: is there a link? *Autoimmun Rev* **2**(2): 69–72.

Sanchez-Borges, M., A. Capriles-Hulett, et al. (2003). Cutaneous reactions to aspirin and nonsteroidal anti-inflammatory drugs. *Clin Rev Allergy Immunol* **24**(2): 125–36.

Stanaland, B. E. (2002). Treatment of patients with chronic idiopathic urticaria. *Clin Rev Allergy Immunol* **23**(2): 233–41.

Wai, Y. C. and G. L. Sussman (2002). Evaluating chronic urticaria patients for allergies, infections, or autoimmune disorders. *Clin Rev Allergy Immunol* **23**(2): 185–93.

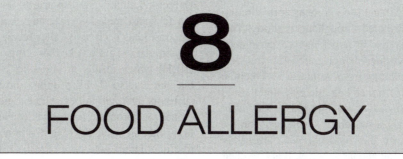

C H A P T E R

8

FOOD ALLERGY

INTRODUCTION

Reactions to food are common, but not all are actually due to allergic mechanisms. There are also abiding myths about food, such as the supposition that there is a link between cow's milk ingestion and mucus production. There are near magical properties that certain beliefs ascribe to foods. For example, there are claims that they will strengthen the immune system or increase intelligence. These beliefs, and a lack of clarity about what constitutes an allergic reaction to food, make it difficult to have an accounting of the actual frequency of true food reactions.

PATHOPHYSIOLOGY

The immunologic mechanisms and responses of the gut have two conflicting demands to meet concurrently. It needs to respond to potential pathogens and other harmful antigens, while remaining unresponsive to large quantities of food antigens. The gut associated lymphoid tissue responds rapidly to a huge array of harmful foreign antigens including major pathogens. There are differences in the migration patterns of gut lymphocytes, but a key response area is in the Peyer's patches located primarily in the distal area of the small intestine. Soluble and particulate antigens are preferentially

taken up through specialized areas of the follicle-associated epithelium at the dome of the Peyer's patch. These specialized cells are known as M cells. Because of their structure, these cells transport soluble and particulate antigens from the lumen to the underlying lymphoid tissue with only minor enzymatic degradation and therefore fully retained antigenicity.

In the Peyer's patch, the primary antigen presenting cell is actually the B cell, which present antigen to T cells via the MHC Class II surface structure. To a lesser extent, macrophages and dendritic cells are also active in presentation of antigen to T cells within the Peyer's patches. T cells proliferate and partially differentiate before migrating through intestinal lymphatics to regional lymph nodes. These cells essentially disseminate the information about the antigen and circulate to the common mucosal lymphoid tissue. The Peyer's patch B cells produce primarily IgA, except in infancy, when they respond with IgM production. The GI tract has other mechanisms that augment the immune response, including the action of a wide range of enzymes and the blocking effect of mucus in the gut. In the young infant, many of these mechanisms are not mature, and there is greater passage of intact antigens into lymphoid tissue, increasing the risk of developing a class switch to IgE and subsequent food allergy.

Mechanism of Development of Food Allergy

Immunologically intact food proteins enter circulation and are distributed throughout the body. This concept was supported by now famous experiments. Prausnitz and Kustner demonstrated the transferability of fish allergy from serum, and Freeman noted that serum from an egg allergy patient could cause local response if it was injected into the nose and the subject subsequently challenged orally. Others have shown that food allergens are easily absorbed from small and large bowel. It is also clear that antigens from the bowel are rapidly disseminated throughout the body to mast in and out of the GI tract.

To prevent an immune response to all ingested foods, there is selectively reduced responsiveness to these antigens. This is a form of tolerance, or, more accurately, hyposensitization. The mechanism is not clear in humans, and most of the studies have been performed in mice and rats. Extrapolating these results to humans is not completely valid, and rodent and human immune responses differ significantly. In general, tolerance is more readily developed in T-cell subsets, than in B cells. Oral ingestion of a protein antigen by a mouse depresses systemic IgM, IgG, and IgE antibody responses. Cell mediated responses to the food are also suppressed. At least in the mouse, CD8+ induced suppression plays a part in the emergence of tolerance, as does the action of antigen presenting cells. Introducing several solid foods in the first 4 months of life in humans increases the likelihood of developing food hypersensitivity. It is probably during the first 4 months that mechanisms emerge that contribute to the ability to develop tolerance. However, it has also been demonstrated in mice that the processing of food antigens by the gut is essential to the development oral tolerance. Some data have even shown that there is a difference in ovalbumin from serum of mice fed ovalbumin, and the serum form has the ability to induce tolerance, and carries B-cell epitopes. Irradiating mice destroys the ability to develop tolerance to ovalbumin, and SCID mice cannot develop tolerance. This indicates that the process is probably dependent on T and B cells. There are few studies of oral tolerance in human subjects. Decreased cutaneous response to an injected hapten (a small molecule that augments an immune response) has been noted after feeding subjects the hapten. An example is keyhole limpet hemocyanin (KLH) which results in systemic T-cell tolerance but can lead to B-cell priming and production of secretory IgA antibodies. The extent of T-cell tolerance was proportional to the dose and immunization schedule used. A generalization is that protective or tolerant antibodies are IgG. Production of IgG to food is universal, and the presence of IgG in serum is not an indicator of an allergy to the food and is not of pathologic significance. High levels of IgE to food are indicative of a potential allergy. It is possible that failure to develop oral tolerance to ingested proteins in human neonates could result in the development of food hypersensitivity. The probability of developing tolerance depends on the type of antigen. For example, tolerance readily develops to soybeans, but development of tolerance to peanuts is rare.

Prospective studies on exclusive breast feeding suggest that there is prevention of food allergy and atopic dermatitis possibly by promoting the development of oral tolerance. Other probable contributing factors to preventing food allergy include decreased exposure to foreign proteins, breast milk sIgA, and induction of the mucosal barrier. In general, the data on the protective effects of breast milk are incomplete, and more studies are needed to draw any firm conclusions. Another consideration, partly supported by other studies, is that high serum levels of food-specific IgG antibodies transferred from mother to fetus before birth are protective against food allergy.

A counter theory suggests that feeding high doses of cow's milk to infants increases CD8+ function, suppressing IgE production. A retrospective analysis of breast-fed infants with a strong family history of atopy suggested that those who were fed significant amounts of cow's milk-based formula in the newborn nursery were less likely to develop atopy by 18 months of age than were those who did not receive supplement. The issues of the protective effects of human milk have not been completely resolved, and there remain open questions regarding whether it prevents allergies, including food allergy.

Causes of Food Allergy

Almost any food has the potential to cause an allergic reaction. However, a few food groups seem to be responsible for most of the reactions. The physicochemical properties that account for the much higher allergenicity of these foods are poorly understood. The following is a discussion of the most frequent causes. Nearly 90% of all food reactions are accounted for by egg, milk, peanut, soybean, and wheat (Table 8-1).

Dairy Products

Cow's milk. Not only is cow's milk the first foreign food protein encountered by infants and a diet staple, it is also most often implicated as causing food reactions. Cow's milk contains at least 20 protein components that have been noted to induce an antibody response. The major milk protein fractions are casein (75%) and whey. Whey contains primarily beta-lactoglobulin, alpha-lactalbumin, bovine immunoglobulins, and bovine serum albumin. Allergy has been described to all of these proteins. From an allergenic point of view, there is considerable cross-reactivity with other animal milk, notably goat's milk. These cannot be substituted for cow's milk in patients who are allergic.

Eggs. Chicken eggs are very common causes of food-allergic reactions in children. The white is more allergenic than the yolk, and some reactions to yolk may be due to contaminating proteins. The major egg white antigen ovomucoid, but the highest concentration is ovalbumin. There is little cross-reactivity with chicken meat, and most egg allergic patients can ingest chicken without problems.

Legumes

Legumes, especially peanuts and soybeans are among the most common food allergens. While the legumes share several antigens, there does not seem to be clinically relevant cross-reactivity.

TABLE 8-1

CAUSES OF FOOD-ALLERGIC REACTIONS

Dairy Products
Cow's milk
Eggs
Legumes
Peanuts
Soybeans
Tree Nuts
Almonds
Brazil nuts
Cashews
Filberts
Pecan
Pine nuts
Pistachios
Walnuts
Fish
Crustacea
Lobsters
Crabs
Prawns
Crayfish
Shrimp
Mollusks
Mussels
Clams
Oysters
Scallops
Snails
Octopus
Squid
Cereal Grains
Wheat
Rye
Barley
Nonfood Proteins
Pollens

Most peanut allergic patients can eat other legumes without risk.

Peanuts. Peanuts are possibly the most allergenic and dangerous food for those who are allergic. There is a high risk for serious reactions, including anaphylaxis. Three proteins have been identified as the major antigens of peanuts (Ara h 1—63.5 kD; Ara h 2—17 kD; Ara h 3—14 kD). Refined peanut oil is generally safe to ingest for allergic people.

Soybeans. This member of the legume family is a significant cause of hypersensitivity reactions predominantly in infants and young children. Soybean protein is used in many commercial foods as a cheap source of high-quality protein. Four allergenic fractions have been identified, and none of them seems to predominate. Refined oil seems safe, but caution should always be advised when a patient is allergic to a product.

Tree Nuts

As a group, nuts are possibly one of the major food allergens in adults. As with peanuts, tree nuts, especially almonds, Brazil nuts, cashews, filberts, pecans, pine nuts, pistachios, and walnuts have been implicated in severe reactions and anaphylaxis. In general, there seems to be considerable cross-sensitivity among tree nuts. Patients allergic to one should be cautious with all common nuts. Peanuts are usually safe, since they are not nuts.

Fish

Edible fish cause a significant number of reactions that can include severe reactions. The major allergen in cod, Gad c 1 (12.3 kD), has been isolated from the myogen fraction. Ten common fish species were shown to have a protein analogous to Gad c 1 that also had immunologic cross-reactivity with codfish. The antigen(s) is susceptible to manipulation and storage, so some patients may react to fresh tuna, but not to canned. It appears that the antigens are easily aerosolized, as patients may develop significant symptoms from the smell of cooking fish. Controversy exists as to whether patients allergic to one species of fish should avoid all.

Crustacea and Mollusks

This group of shellfish is a major allergen possibly affecting up to 250,000 adults in the United States. Crustacea include lobsters, crabs, prawns, crayfish, and shrimp. Mollusks comprise three classes that include mussels, clams, oysters, scallops, snails, octopus, and squid among them.

Shrimp contains several allergens. Antigen II was believed to be the major allergen from the shell. Shrimp muscle glycoprotein contains Pen a 1 (tropomyosin). There is considerable cross-reactivity among the crustacea.

Cereal Grains

Cereals are relatively frequent, especially in children, as a cause for an allergic reaction. The globulin and glutenin fractions seem to be major allergenic fractions in IgE-mediated reactions, while gliadins are the cause of celiac disease. There is extensive cross-reactivity among wheat, rye, and barley. Positive prick skin tests are common among children, but the clinical significance must be interpreted in the context of reactions to ingested cereals. New varieties of rice and other cereals have been produced with reduced allergenic activity by use of genetic engineering. Patients sensitized to airborne psyllium (a component of commercial bulk laxatives) developed anaphylactic reactions upon ingestion of a cereal containing psyllium. In adults, especially working in bakeries, there is a risk of sensitization and development of rhinitis and asthma from inhalation of flour dust. Surprisingly, many of these patients can ingest wheat products.

Contaminating Nonfood Proteins

Pollens and other inedible contaminants have been described as sources of cross-reaction with foods. These reactions occur in both directions: patients allergic to hazelnuts can react to birch pollen, and patients allergic to birch may develop symptoms on eating hazelnuts.

Common cross-reactions that have been described include the following:

> *Birch pollen*: apples, raw potatoes, carrots, celery, and hazelnuts
> *Mugwort (a weed) pollen*: celery, apple, peanut, and kiwifruit

Ragweed pollen: melons

Latex: bananas, avocado, kiwifruit, chestnut, and papaya

CLINICAL

From a clinical and management point of view, it is important to distinguish reactions that are mediated by IgE from those that have other mechanisms.

There are three main types of reaction to food: allergic, sensitivity, and toxin related. The key features of theses are shown in Table 8-2.

True allergic reactions are those that are mediated by IgE. The signs and symptoms are due to release of histamine, leukotrienes, prostaglandins, and cytokines, as with any other allergic reaction. There are key features that help to distinguish this type of reaction from others.

The onset of an allergic response is within 30 minutes of ingestion of the food. There is a loose correlation between the degree of allergy to a food and the rapidity of onset of a clinical reaction to it. A patient who is highly allergic to a food may have an onset of symptoms within minutes or even seconds of ingestion. A second feature of an allergic reaction is apparent dose independence. This result in as severe a reaction to very small quantities of the antigen as would occur with a large dose. Thus, a patient may develop anaphylaxis to a peanut touching the lip as readily as to eating a large quantity of peanuts. The reason for this phenomenon is that a titration curve for foods occurs in the microgram to milligram dose range and is then flat over further increases in concentration. In highly allergic patients, the microgram concentrations contain more

TABLE 8-2

SUMMARY OF THE CHARACTERISTICS OF THREE TYPES OF REACTION TO FOODS, ALLERGY, SENSITIVITY, AND TOXIC REACTIONS

Reaction	Mechanism	Onset	Dose
Allergy	IgE	<30 minutes	Independent
Sensitivity	Idiosyncrasy	Variable	Titration
Toxin	Chemical	Hours	Titration

than adequate protein to cause a severe reaction. Another characteristic of an allergic reaction is rapid involvement of multiple sites and organs.

Sensitivity reactions are not mediated by IgE but some are regulated by IgG. An example is the sensitivity to gliadin, a major protein of wheat, that occurs in sprue and related diseases. In this situation, the patient presents with fat malabsorption and steatorrhea as a result of an immune reaction between IgG antibodies to gliadin and wheat. The reaction takes place in the mucosal surface, leading to flattening of the microvilli and malabsorption. In general, the patient who is having a sensitivity reaction has an exaggerated normal response to a food or food additive. An example is a reaction to caffeine, where some people have sleeplessness after ingestion of a small quantity of coffee or other source of caffeine. Another common confounder is lactose intolerance, which can be confused with milk allergy, especially in infants. In contrast to a true allergy, the reaction is dose dependent and there is a direct correlation between the amount ingested and the patient's reaction. The reaction has a variable onset, from within a few minutes to a few hours of exposure.

Toxic reactions are caused by irritants or poisons in the food, for example mushrooms, contaminated milk, and meat or pesticide residues tainting food. These reactions can have an onset from a few hours to a day or even longer, especially if the toxin has a cumulative effect. There is a good correlation between dose and degree of reaction. Where systemic effects are seen, they are those of sepsis, or the effects of a toxin.

An intriguing question is why an ingested allergen produces widespread effects. The pattern of response, such as urticaria, is determined by random distribution of IgE on mast cells throughout the body. The food is partly digested. In the small bowel there is direct absorption of peptides at sites of Peyer's patches. The Peyer's patches are covered by thin-walled cells, termed M cells, that allow the passage of peptides directly into the Peyer's patches. Once in the geminal center of the Peyer's patch, the antigen can bind with follicular dendritic cells and Langerhans cells. These cells have the ability to migrate through the lymphatics, disseminating information about the antigen. This is one mechanism for skin accumulation of specific IgE. On subsequent exposure the antigen may migrate directly into lymphatics and cause diffuse reactions.

The essential elements of an antigen that trigger an immune response are termed epitopes. An epitope can be as small as a few amino acids, provided that they maintain the essential quaternary three-dimensional shape that is recognized by the antibody. The Fab portion of the immunoglobulin primarily recognizes the three-dimensional shape of the antigen. Thus, only a small fragment of the protein may be needed to bind with IgE, and even digested protein can cause a reaction.

Allergic reactions to food are common. Not all reactions are the result of an IgE-mediated reaction.

Sensitivity

There are many examples of chemicals that can cause sensitivity reactions that can be confused with a true IgE-mediated allergic reaction. The types of sensitivity are noted in Table 8-3.

Toxins

Toxic products in food can cause reactions that can be confused with allergic responses. These can be chemical in nature or due to growth of organisms in the food.

Typical examples are given in Table 8-4.

True Allergic Reactions

Clinical Presentation

True allergic reactions to food have limited manifestations. There are three main areas of presentation: gastrointestinal, skin, and respiratory.

Upper airway. The primary site of contact with the offending antigen is the mouth and lips, and this is usually the first reaction following exposure to the offending antigen. There may be a complaint of itching of the mouth and throat or swelling of the lips and tongue. There is a risk that the patient may

TABLE 8-3

DIFFERENT MECHANISMS OF FOOD SENSITIVITIES WITH EXAMPLES OF EACH

Mechanism	Category	Examples
Intolerance	Sugars	Lactose
		Sucrose
		Mannose
	Alcohol	Beer
		Wine
		Spirits
	Caffeine	Coffee
		Soft drinks
Chemical	Sodium metabisulfite	Salads
		Wine
		Dried fruit
	Monosodium glutamate	Chinese food
	Nitrites	Preservatives
	Nitrates	Meat, fish
	Histamine	Fish
		Cabbage
	Phenylethylamine	Chocolate
	Serotonin	Banana
		Tomato
	Theobromine	Chocolate
		Tea
	Tryptamine	Tomato
		Plum
	Tyramine	Aged cheeses
		Red wine
		Some pickled food
Cross-Reactions	Azo dyes	Tartrazine

Note: Subcategories are shown in the central column.

develop laryngeal edema, with the danger of respiratory arrest.

Gastrointestinal. Among the frequent symptoms are gastrointestinal cramping, emesis, nausea and diarrhea. There is often rapid onset after ingestion of the food, sometimes within minutes.

Skin. Urticaria, angioedema, eczema.

TABLE 8-4

MECHANISMS OF TOXIC REACTIONS

Mechanism	Category	Example
Toxins	Bacterial	Clostridium botulinum
		Staphylococcus aureus
		Salmonella
		Shigella
		Escherichia coli
		Yersinia
		Campylobacter
	Fungal	Aflatoxins
		Trichothecium toxins
		Ergot
Poisons	Scrombroid	Tuna
		Mackerel
		Improperly cleaned wood cutting boards
	Ciguatera	Grouper
		Snapper
		Barracuda
	Saxitoxin	Shellfish
	Heavy metals	Mercury
		Copper
	Pesticides	
Infections	Virus	Hepatitis viruses
		Rotavirus
		Enterovirus
	Parasites	Giardia
		Trichinella

Mechanisms of toxic reactions are presented in the left hand column. Subcategories with examples of each are noted in the table.

Anaphylaxis

IgE-Mediated Hypersensitivity

Gastrointestinal Food Hypersensitivity Reactions

Mechanism. There is a sharp increase in gastric acid secretion, delayed gastric emptying, and mast cell degranulation with a rise in intraluminal histamine. Na^+, Cl^-, and water absorption decrease sharply and bowel contractility increases leading to diarrhea. There is significant disruption of the basement membrane. However, the mucosal architecture appears largely unchanged after a reaction.

In humans, as has been shown in rats, repeated ingestion of a food allergen resulted in the emergence of chronic inflammation, but no acute symptoms. An extended period of complete food allergen avoidance enhances a distinctive response to oral food challenges. Following oral ingestion of a food allergen, there is a combination of hypertonicity in the transverse and pelvic colon and hypotonicity in the cecum and ascending colon. Gastric retention and colonic spasm also occur. The gastric mucosa becomes markedly hyperemic and edematous, with patches of thick gray mucus and scattered petechiae.

Gastrointestinal tract

Oral syndrome: This is a form of contact allergy primarily occurring in the oropharynx. Other sites are rarely involved.

Symptoms include the rapid onset of pruritus and angioedema of the lips, tongue, palate, and throat. The symptoms often follow a pattern of rapid resolution of symptoms. The usual antigens are derived from various fresh fruits and vegetables. There is commonly a history of allergic rhinitis due to birch or ragweed pollens. There may be cross-reaction with fruits and vegetables as noted above. The diagnosis is usually confirmed by prick skin test. It should be kept in mind that the pollen allergy is often the primary problem.

Therapy with antihistamines will provide relief of symptoms. The patient should be observed, at least after initial therapy to ensure that these are not initial symptoms of a systemic reaction.

Gastrointestinal symptoms: Following ingestion of an allergen, gastrointestinal symptoms generally develop within minutes to 2 hours of consumption, but will generally occur within 30 minutes. The key manifestations are nausea, abdominal pain, cramps, and vomiting with or without diarrhea. The duration is usually self-limited. The cause is often local edema and sudden release of allergic mediators.

The diagnosis is established by clinical history and prick skin testing. Complete elimination of the suspected food allergen for up to 2 weeks should produce resolution of symptoms. If food challenges are performed, they should confirm the food as a cause of the symptoms.

Allergic eosinophilic syndromes

Gastroenteritis: Eosinophilic infiltrates can be found in the stomach, esophagus, and proximal small bowel. Eosinophilic infiltration primarily into the stomach is most often associated with allergies, but esophagus and small bowel are usually involved as well. Vasculitis is not a feature, and there is peripheral eosinophilia in about 50% of patients. Infiltration can be under the serosa, in which case there is associated ascites containing eosinophils.

Presentation is commonly with postprandial nausea and vomiting, abdominal pain, and diarrhea. Occasionally there is fat malabsorption manifesting as steatorrhea. Weight loss and failure to thrive may be present. Allergy as an etiology is associated with mucosal infiltrates and not involvement of the deep layers of mucosa. There is also associated elevated IgE in duodenal fluids, other atopic diseases, elevated serum IgE concentrations and positive skin prick tests to a variety of foods and inhalant antigens. There may also be peripheral blood eosinophilia and iron-deficiency anemia.

This is a biopsy diagnosis in patients with suspect symptoms. Since the eosinophilic infiltrates may be patchy, biopsies may be needed from up to eight sites. Supportive features include the presence of peripheral eosinophilia and Charcot-Leyden crystals (from eosinophils) in the stools. Serum IgE concentration is often elevated and allergy skin tests may be positive. Tests for malabsorption, such as D-xylose may be depressed. The final diagnosis is made by elimination of the responsible food allergen with resolution of symptoms and eosinophilic infiltrate.

Infantile colic: Infantile colic is poorly defined, but usual features include fussiness, intense paroxysms of crying, drawing up of the legs and excessive gas. It generally develops in the first 2–4 weeks of life and persists through the third to fourth month of life. In about 10–15% of colicky infants, food allergy may be a contributing cause. If an allergy is suspected as the cause, the diagnosis can be supported by using a hypoallergenic formula (such as Alimentum) and should recur when the regular formula is reintroduced. Periodic rechallenges should be performed every 3–4 months.

Respiratory symptoms

Rhinitis: A commonly held myth is that "milk makes mucus" and that ingestion of milk products is associated with nasal congestion. In fact, studies show that only 0.08–0.2% of infants develop nasal symptoms after oral milk challenge. Even in older children, the perception of rhinitis that improves after milk is withdrawn from the diet (20%) is only sustained by double-blind food challenge in 0.6% of children. In some infants who have cow's milk allergy associated with high serum IgE, the presenting symptom is often rhinitis. From a clinical standpoint, food allergens are rarely an aggravating factor in chronic rhinoconjunctivitis and asthma, even though there is evidence that food antigens can provoke airway hyperreactivity.

Pulmonary: In a broader sense, food allergies and exposure to allergenic foods can aggravate respiratory symptoms. In several studies as many as 39% of children with positive blinded food challenge had respiratory symptoms that included sneezing, rhinorrhea, nasal obstruction, wheezing and cough, and laryngeal symptoms that may include tightness in the throat and a staccato cough.

Pulmonary symptoms associated with the ingestion to food may include a sensation of chest tightness or shortness of breath, deep cough, or wheezing. The distribution of symptoms in one study was nasal symptoms, 63%; laryngeal symptoms, 43%; and pulmonary symptoms, 24%.

The types of food that initiate respiratory symptoms are predominantly fish and shrimp. These antigens can provoke an immediate pulmonary reaction, with nasal symptoms occurring in anywhere from 30 to 80%. Symptoms typically developed within 15–90 minutes of initiation of the challenge and lasted from 30 to 120 minutes. Nasal fluid histamine and eosinophil cationic protein (ECP) were found to increase significantly in children experiencing nasal symptoms. About 15% of patients with food allergy develop pulmonary symptoms, including chest tightness, cough, and wheezing during a food challenge. A much lower number, about 7.5%, experienced a fall in forced expiratory volume in 1 second (FEV1). Food-induced bronchospasm has been found in 8.5% of a cohort of asthmatic children. A greater than a twofold decrease in methacholine-inhalation challenge PD20 FEV1 was noted comparing results before and after a food challenge. The frequency seems to be higher in children than in adults.

The diagnosis of food-induced airway disease should be considered in patients with a history of food-induced wheezing or in asthmatics who are refractory to medication.

Skin Reactions

Some of the more dramatic reactions to food begin in the skin. They are certainly the most noticed by the patients and parents. They are probably the most common reactions to foods.

Urticaria and angioedema. The prevalence of these reactions is unknown, but estimates place them at 20–40% of the general population. The frequency is higher in children. (See chapter on Urticaria and Angioedema for details.) Considering that the onset of symptoms often follows within minutes of ingestion of the responsible allergen, the cause is often not known. Multiple foods may be ingested simultaneously or soon after each other. The onset may also be delayed, but usually not beyond 30 minutes. The foods most commonly incriminated in children: eggs, milk, peanuts, and nuts. In adults, the usual causes are fish, shellfish, nuts, and peanuts. Food is generally involved in acute urticaria, but in chronic urticaria food is not usually identified as a cause.

Atopic dermatitis. There is controversy regarding the role of food allergy in the genesis of atopic dermatitis. There are data that indicate that one-third of children seen in an allergy clinic had food allergy contributing to their skin symptoms. The degree of severity of atopic dermatitis has also been correlated with increased food hypersensitivity. There is a stronger correlation with repeated ingestion of the offending food, rather than an acute exposure. A large series indicated skin reactions in 75% of

patients challenged orally. These reactions resembled atopic dermatitis rather than urticaria. Following oral challenge, patients can have gastrointestinal symptoms, upper respiratory symptoms, and wheeze.

An oral challenge will induce immediate and late phase effects on skin and upper airway.

Pathophysiologic changes following oral challenge. There is an increase in activated eosinophils (hypodense) eosinophils in the peripheral blood. Eosinophils infiltrate at the site of the lesions. Plasma histamine concentration rises in proportion to the response to challenge. When the antigen is chronically ingested, there is also a rise in histamine releasing factor that is spontaneously released by mononuclear cells. This level falls over time when the food is withdrawn. At the same time, there is no change in basophil number in circulation or in the levels of complement products, C3a or C5a in plasma.

Anaphylaxis

Food-induced anaphylaxis. Food allergy is the most common cause of anaphylaxis seen in hospital emergency departments, accounting for about one-third of the cases. Insect stings were the next common, causing 15% of the reactions. There are about 100 fatal cases of food-induced anaphylaxis in the United States each year. The usual presentation includes cutaneous, respiratory, and gastrointestinal symptoms of food allergy, with the addition of hypotension, vascular collapse, and dysrhythmias. A review of fatal episodes of anaphylaxis showed several common features. All had asthma, and had unknowingly ingested the food allergen. They had previously had allergic reactions to the food, and the onset of symptoms was within minutes of ingestion. The patients who died had not received epinephrine immediately, or used an EpiPen. Where epinephrine was used immediately, it prevented acute fatality, but not necessarily severe morbidity. This supports the concept that the use of epinephrine (EpiPen) by the patient or parent must be immediately followed by emergency room care.

Exercise-induced anaphylaxis. This is a rare form of anaphylaxis. It occurs only when exercise follows the ingestion of a food to which the patient is allergic. The patient exercises within 3–4 hours after ingesting the food. Two forms of food-dependent exercise-induced anaphylaxis have been described: reactions after the ingestion of specific foods and rarely reactions after the ingestion of any food. If the patient ingests the food without exercise, no reactions occur. The condition is associated with asthma and other atopic disorders, and skin prick tests are often positive. Females are affected twice as often as in males. Foods that have been implicated include wheat, fish and shellfish, fruit, milk, and celery. The management involves avoidance of the food. Immediate management includes having adrenalin and an antihistamine available.

Airborne food allergens. Many food-allergic patients may react during cooking, or other means of aerosolizing the antigen, as with people chewing peanuts. Other common causes include fish, mollusks, crustacea, and eggs. It is advisable for severely allergic patients to exert caution when around food that may become aerosolized.

Non-IgE-Mediated Food Hypersensitivity

Gastrointestinal Food Hypersensitivity

Celiac disease. This condition is an extensive enteropathy leading to malabsorption. The incidence is reported as 1 of 4000 but may be as high as 1/300 in some populations. The cause is sensitivity to gliadin, which is a strongly antigenic portion of gluten. Gluten is found in wheat, oat, rye, and barley. The result of ingestion is that there is total villous atrophy and extensive cellular infiltrate into the lamina propria. The patients have high levels of IgA directed against gliadin. When wheat is ingested, an immune complex reaction occurs in the mucosa and submucosa of small bowel. Symptoms often include diarrhea or frank steatorrhea, abdominal distension and flatulence, weight loss, and occasionally nausea and vomiting.

Pathophysiology. Ninety percent of patients with celiac disease are HLA-B8-positive, and nearly 80% have the HLA-Dw3 antigen. Villous atrophy

of the small bowel is a characteristic feature of celiac patients after ingesting gluten and there is a prominent infiltrate with CD8+ cytotoxic/suppressor cells. There is an increase in IgM- and IgA-containing B cells. Serum IgA is increased, with specific antibodies to gliadin. IgA antibodies to gluten are present in over 80% of adults and children with untreated celiac disease. Cellular Type IV mechanisms are prominent in the pathology. Serum concentrations of immune complexes do correlate well with disease activity.

Diagnosis. The diagnosis is based on a challenge-rechallenge procedure. Following biopsy evidence of villous atrophy and inflammatory infiltrate (required for diagnosis) gluten is withdrawn from the diet for 6–12 weeks. The patient is then rechallenged with gluten with recurrence of biopsy changes. Titers of IgA antigliadin antibodies may be used for screening with IgA antiendomysium antibodies and possibly antijejunal antibodies in patients over 2 years of age.

Therapy. Therapy consists of total life-long elimination of gluten-containing foods. One long-term risk of continued gluten ingestion is the development of bowel malignancy.

Enterocolitis syndrome. This is a disorder of young infants, mostly between 1 week and 3 months of age. The infants present with protracted vomiting and diarrhea. Cow's milk and soybean protein are most often responsible.

Clinical presentation is mainly with vomiting and diarrhea within 1–3 hours of ingestion. Shock may occur in about 15% of cases. Adults may develop a similar picture, but less severe, to seafood. Stools often contain occult blood, polymorphonuclear neutrophils, and eosinophils and frequently show the presence of reducing substances from malabsorbed sugars. Skin prick tests are characteristically negative. Jejunal biopsy specimens classically reveal flattened villi, edema, and increased numbers of lymphocytes, eosinophils, and mast cells. The cause of this syndrome remains unknown. Food challenge will confirm the diagnosis, but should only be performed in a setting where assistance is immediately available.

Eosinophilic colitis. Presentation is in the first few months of life. The cause is cow's milk or soybean protein hypersensitivity. Cases can occur in breast-fed infants. The children are asymptomatic, and present with blood loss, occasionally leading to anemia.

Diagnosis is based on a response to avoiding the food. Symptoms then resolve within 72 hours.

Enteropathy. This is a group of non-IgE-mediated allergic responses that presents in the first several months of life with diarrhea or even steatorrhea. Failure to thrive is prominent. Cow's milk sensitivity is the most frequent cause of this syndrome. It also occurs with sensitivity to soybeans, eggs, wheat, rice, chicken, and fish. IgA and IgG antibodies specific to cow's milk proteins are elevated. Therapy consists of identifying the causative food and eliminating it.

Pulmonary
Hemosiderosis (Heiner's Syndrome)

There is controversy regarding whether this syndrome of recurrent episodes of pneumonia associated with pulmonary infiltrates, hemosiderosis, gastrointestinal blood loss, and iron-deficiency anemia is truly related to reactions to cow's milk. The diagnosis is supported by finding hemosiderin-laden macrophages from early morning gastric aspirates or from lung biopsy. Elimination of milk and egg proteins from the diet is associated with resolution of the condition. The presence of characteristic laboratory data, including precipitating antibodies to cow's milk and in vitro proliferation of T cells to cow's milk antigen support the diagnosis.

Dermatitis Herpetiformis

This condition is often mistaken for atopic dermatitis. The rash is intensely pruritic and is associated with gluten-sensitive enteropathy. The papulovesicular rash is symmetrically distributed over the extensor surfaces. About 85% of patients have gluten enteropathy, and a high percentage have HLA-B8. Skin biopsy demonstrates granular deposit of IgA.

Sulfones produce rapid resolution of pruritus and a response of the skin lesions, but have no effect on celiac-like gastrointestinal features.

Other Conditions Linked to Food

Gustatory rhinitis. In this condition, patients develop rhinorrhea following the ingestion of chili peppers. The reaction is cholinergic and is inhibited by anticholinergic agents. The active ingredient causing the reaction is probably capsaicin.

Inflammatory bowel disease. There is little evidence to convincingly link Crohn's disease and ulcerative colitis with cow's milk allergy.

Behavior. Hyperactivity and attention deficit disorder have been associated with a variety of food "reactions." There is little scientific basis for this link. Patients suffering from sleep deprivation because of nasal obstruction or asthma symptoms may have secondary attention or behavior problems.

There is also little evidence to support that eating sugar-containing foods or dyes or salicylate like substances causes "hyperactivity." There is also little evidence to support fad diets, such as the Feingold diet, in the management of hyperactivity disorders.

Arthritis. There is only anecdotal suggestion that arthritis is worsened by particular foods. Blinded food challenge studies do not bear this out and there are no scientific studies that support this contention.

Central nervous system

Migraines. True migraine headaches can be triggered by foods that contain tyramines and other specific monoamines. However, there are few studies with data to link them to food allergies.

Seizures. Some studies using blinded challenge have implicated food allergies as triggers for seizures. These data need confirmation.

Autism. The assertion has been made that food allergies contribute to the emergence of autism. There are no scientific data to link autism and related syndromes to food allergy.

Sudden infant death syndrome. This is a condition in which an infant, usually aged 2–4 months is found dead in a crib. No reason is apparent, despite intensive research. Some studies have indicated that there is an increase in tryptase in serum in these infants. Tryptase is an indicator of recent mast cell activation, and may suggest that anaphylaxis has occurred. These infants may have IgE antibodies directed against beta-lactoglobulin, raising the suspicion of milk allergy as a cause of anaphylaxis and death in these infants. Further confirmation is needed.

APPROACH TO DIAGNOSIS

History

Onset

The history is most helpful in food reactions, especially since there is a narrow temporal relationship between exposure and the onset of the reaction. Most acute food reactions occur within minutes, but there may be a delay up to 30 minutes. This limits the time-frame that the patient has to consider (Table 8-5).

Pattern

The pattern of lesions is not usually specific or helpful. Contact reactions tend to start at the site of contact. People who handle shrimp and are allergic to them will have lesions that start on the hands.

Helpful Features in the History Include the Following:

A presumption of the responsible food from the parent or patient
Previous reaction to the food
Quantity of food ingested
Associated factors
Interval between ingestion and development of symptoms
The presence of cofactors, such as exercise
Time interval since last reaction
The history is only as reliable as the patient's or parent's recall of the events. Other methods have been tried to augment the detection of allergies

TABLE 8-5

AN OVERVIEW OF THE APPROACH TO DIAGNOSIS OF FOOD ALLERGIES

History
  Onset
  Pattern
    Previous reaction
    Quantity of food
    Associated factors
  Diet diaries
  Elimination diets

Investigation
  Skin prick tests
  Intradermal
    Not recommended for foods
  Radioallergosorbent tests (RASTs)
  Double-blind placebo-controlled food challenge
    The "gold standard"

Unproven diagnostic tests
  Food-specific IgG or IgG4 antibody levels
  Food antigen-antibody complexes
  Lymphocyte activation
  Sublingual or intracutaneous provocation

Note: discussed in the text.

Monitoring

Diet diaries. The use of a diary is helpful as it removes the need for recall. The patient is asked to record food intake at each meal for a set period, usually 2–4 weeks. The patient or parent then annotates the entries with comments regarding allergic reactions. This way, a pattern of reaction to food or combinations of food becomes obvious. The problem with this approach is the obvious one that most diaries are poorly kept. If the patient is meticulous, however, this is a very helpful tool.

Elimination diets. This is a direct approach to augment the history. Suspected foods are scrupulously avoided. The patient notes whether symptoms improve. An easy example is the infant suspected of having cow's milk allergy can be placed on Alimentum or another elemental formula that contains only amino acids. Symptoms can then be monitored.

The situation is more complex with the older child or adult. It is not easy to completely avoid a common antigen, such as wheat or peanuts. This problem is compounded if the disease has a more subtle or even controversial relationship with food, as is the case in atopic dermatitis or asthma. Thus, elimination diets alone rarely confirm the diagnosis of food allergy.

Investigation

Skin Prick Tests

Skin prick tests can be performed in a standard manner (see Investigation of Allergies). Positive skin tests are weak, as the overall positive predictive value is 50–65%. This test must be correlated with history. On the other hand, a negative test carries a 95% negative predictive value. This is helpful to exclude foods as a cause of the symptoms.

For instance, a patient who suspects that he/she has an allergy to shrimp can be reassured by a negative prick skin test. The accuracy of the test is proportional to the purity of the antigen in the test extract. Where there is disagreement between the skin test and history, the decision should favor the history, especially if there is a strong clinical response with a negative allergy test. The test should be repeated with fresh antigen.

Intradermal

Intradermal testing is not recommended for foods. There is an even higher rate of false positives, and there is a serious risk of the patient having an allergic reaction.

Radioallergosorbent Tests (RASTs)

The RAST and related assays are less sensitive than skin testing, but the same limitations apply in interpretation. A negative is more meaningful than a positive. If there is a risk of severe reaction, the RAST is safer than a skin test. In general, in vitro measurements of serum food-specific IgE performed in high-quality laboratories provide information

similar to that of skin prick tests. The test is useful in young children, in those with dermographism and those with severe skin disease.

The "Gold Standard"

The double-blind placebo-controlled food challenge (DBPCFC) has been used successfully in food allergy. The selection of foods to be tested in DBPCFCs is generally based upon history or skin test (RAST) results. Suspected foods should be eliminated for 7–14 days before challenge. Antihistamines should be discontinued long enough to establish a normal histamine skin test, and other medications should be minimized to levels sufficient to prevent breakthrough of acute symptoms. In asthmatic patients FEV1 should be maintained >70% predicted value before challenging. Short bursts of corticosteroids may be necessary to meet these criteria.

The food challenge is administered in the fasting state, starting with a dose unlikely to provoke symptoms (25–500 mg of lyophilized food). The dose is then doubled every 15–60 minutes, depending on the type of reaction suspected. In a negative test, the patient tolerates 10 g of lyophilized food blinded in capsules or liquid. If the blinded challenge is negative, however, it must be confirmed by an open feeding under observation to rule out the rare false-negative challenge. An equal number of food antigen and placebo challenges should be used. Overall, this is a very precise tool for confirming food allergy.

Unproven Diagnostic Tests

There is no clinical evidence to support the use of food-specific IgG or IgG4 antibody levels, food antigen-antibody complexes, evidence of lymphocyte activation or sublingual or intracutaneous provocation. These tests have little value when tested in a controlled manner.

THERAPY

Avoidance

Essentially, the therapy of food allergy is the avoidance of the food. This can be difficult to achieve. Consultation with a nutritionist is useful for the

TABLE 8-6

OVERVIEW OF THE ESSENTIAL THERAPY OF FOOD ALLERGY

Avoidance

Medication

  Epinephrine

    Epinephrine 1/1000 w/v—0.01 mL/kg to a
      maximum of 0.5 mL

    EpiPen 0.15 and 0.3 mL of 1/1000 w/v solution

Antihistamines

  Diphenhydramine

  Hydroxyzine

Steroids

  Solu-Medrol

    50–100 mg immediately

    1 mg/kg to a maximum of 80 mg daily for 5 days

Prevention

  Gastrocrom

  Xolair

Note: Avoidance is the major therapeutic approach.

patient to develop a menu that eliminates the food and still remains nutritious. Some foods are ubiquitous and difficult to avoid completely, such as wheat or soy. There are several web sites that can help the patient with dependable advice and recipes. The Food Allergy Network (http://www.foodallergy.org/index.html), the American Academy of Allergy, Asthma and Immunology (http://www.aaaai.org/) and the American College of Allergy, Asthma and Immunology (http://allergy.mcg.edu/) are excellent sites for reliable information (Table 8-6).

Medication

Epinephrine

The immediate treatment of an acute episode should be the use of epinephrine, 1/1000 w/v solution at a dose of 0.01 mL/kg to a maximum of 0.5 mL. It is injected subcutaneously. Recent studies have indicated that the intramuscular route may be preferable.

Patients who have had a potentially life-threatening episode, or may be at risk for such an episode, need to have epinephrine immediately available. The easiest form that is currently available is EpiPen, which an automatically injecting syringe. The patient removes the cap and presses the end against the fleshy part of the thigh. There is no need to waste time removing clothing. There are two strengths, 0.15 and 0.3 mL of 1/1000 w/v solution.

Antihistamines

Diphenhydramine or hydroxyzine, 25–50 mg should be given immediately and then tid to qid for 4–5 days depending on the response.

Steroids

Patients who have respiratory involvement should be given Solu-Medrol 50–100 mg immediately and then 1 mg/kg to a maximum of 80 mg daily for 5 days. The initial dose should be given intravenously if the patient has respiratory difficulties. IV fluids and hospitalization are indicated if the patient has a fall in blood pressure or is shocked.

Prevention

Cromolyn

The use of Gastrocrom, 100–200 mg qid is useful in reducing the reaction to allergenic foods.

Xolair

This is a monoclonal antibody directed against IgE. Its use in food allergy has had limited study, but an investigation in patients with severe reactions to peanuts showed that they had increased tolerance following a course of the biological agent. It is given as an intramuscular injection once to twice per month. The drug is extremely expensive, and an annual cost can be higher than $10,000.

SUMMARY

Food reactions are complex. The diagnosis remains a clinical exercise dependent on a careful history, selective allergy tests if an IgE-mediated disorder is suspected and an appropriate exclusion diet

Suggested Reading

Al-Muhsen, S., A. E. Clarke, et al. (2003). Peanut allergy: an overview. *CMAJ* **168**(10): 1279–85.

Bahna, S. L. (2003). Clinical expressions of food allergy. *Ann Allergy Asthma Immunol* **90**(6 Suppl. 3): 41–4.

Bahna, S. L. (2003). Diagnosis of food allergy. *Ann Allergy Asthma Immunol* **90**(6 Suppl. 3): 77–80.

Bernstein, J. A., I. L. Bernstein, et al. (2003). Clinical and laboratory investigation of allergy to genetically modified foods. *Environ Health Perspect* **111**(8): 1114–21.

Bock, S. A. (2003). Diagnostic evaluation. *Pediatrics* **111**(6 Pt. 3): 1638–44.

Burks, W. (2003). Skin manifestations of food allergy. *Pediatrics* **111**(6 Pt. 3): 1617–24.

Crespo, J. F. and J. Rodriguez (2003). Food allergy in adulthood. *Allergy* **58**(2): 98–113.

Eigenmann, P. A. (2002). T lymphocytes in food allergy: overview of an intricate network of circulating and organ-resident cells. *Pediatr Allergy Immunol* **13**(3): 162–71.

Hubbard, S. (2003). Nutrition and food allergies: the dietitian's role. *Ann Allergy Asthma Immunol* **90**(6 Suppl. 3): 115–6.

Sampson, H. A. (2003). 9. Food allergy. *J Allergy Clin Immunol* **111**(2 Suppl.): S540–7.

Sampson, H. A. (2003). The evaluation and management of food allergy in atopic dermatitis. *Clin Dermatol* **21**(3): 183–92.

Sicherer, S. H. (2003). Advances in anaphylaxis and hypersensitivity reactions to foods, drugs, and insect venom. *J Allergy Clin Immunol* **111**(3 Suppl.): S829–34.

Tang, A. W. (2003). A practical guide to anaphylaxis. *Am Fam Physician* **68**(7): 1325–32.

Teuber, S. S. and C. Porch-Curren (2003). Unproved diagnostic and therapeutic approaches to food allergy and intolerance. *Curr Opin Allergy Clin Immunol* **3**(3): 217–21.

Wuthrich, B. (1998). Food-induced cutaneous adverse reactions. *Allergy* **53**(46 Suppl.): 131–5.

AN APPROACH TO THE WHEEZING INFANT

THE PROBLEM OF WHEEZING IN INFANCY

Despite being frequently noted in infants, wheezing is actually an unhelpful sign.

It indicates only that there is an obstruction causing turbulence in the airways, without suggesting the location of the obstruction, the severity, or its cause. This is especially true in infants. Normal airflow is laminar in the airways, and there is a direct relationship between pressure and airflow (Figure 9-1). Laminar flow is nearly silent. If there is an obstruction in the airway, or outside compressing a bronchus, laminar flow breaks up and airflow becomes audible as a wheeze. The relationship of flow and pressure change, and the square of the pressure is now needed to maintain the same flow rate.

An important clinical paradox is that the patient has to maintain a reasonable airflow rate to generate a wheeze. If the patient is tiring or severely obstructed, they cannot move enough air to wheeze because of the marked increase in pressure requirements. These flow mechanics are even more marked in a small infant, whose airways are narrower at baseline. For these reasons, it is important to consider the broad differential diagnosis in small infants presenting with wheeze.

Case Presentation

These two similar scenarios represent the essential problem of an infant who has wheezing.

1. An 8-month-old male who presents with
   - Cough and wheeze for 2 weeks
   - First presentation
2. Eight-month-old male
   - Cough, wheeze for 2 weeks
   - Third presentation

In the first instance, the cause is likely to be an acute viral infection, especially a pulmonary inflammatory virus, such as respiratory syncytial virus (RSV) or adenovirus.

Explanation

In case 2, there is a recurrent element, with implied reversibility. This raises many other possibilities, including asthma and mechanical processes. These considerations are not always easy to sort out, and it is not always obvious which infant may develop asthma or have wheezing that is postviral and resolves.

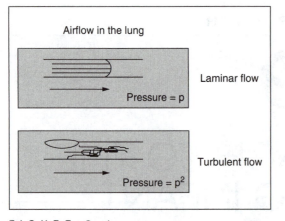

FIGURE 9-1

AIRFLOW IN THE LUNG.

Airflow in the lung is represented by the two diagrams in this figure. The top diagram demonstrates laminar flow. In this mode, which is the normal unobstructed flow, there is a direct relationship between pressure in the airways and flow rate. The lower diagram indicates the breakup of laminar flow that occurs in turbulent flow. Turbulent flow is caused by a partial obstruction to the lumen, as occurs in asthma. This turbulent flow is heard as a wheeze clinically. In this mode the flow rate is proportional to the square of the pressure exerted in the airways. This means that a patient with partially obstructed airways must exert a far higher pressure in the airways to maintain the same flow as occurs in the laminar flow state. This phenomenon is experienced as breathlessness by the patient.

DIFFERENTIAL CONSIDERATIONS IN THE WHEEZING INFANT

There is a large differential diagnosis to consider for the infant who presents with wheezing. Wheezing is common under 1 year of age and may be due to transient mechanical problems or may be the first indicator of a long-term disease process.

The source of wheeze can be from the upper, middle, or lower respiratory tract. These causes are listed in Table 9-1.

The common conditions on the list in Table 9-1 that frequently occur in infancy and should be considered include the following:

Asthma

This condition is discussed in Chap. 6. It is difficult to diagnose this condition under the age of 6 months. In general, other causes should be excluded, and the patient given a trial of bronchodilator therapy. A good response to albuterol indicates reversibility of the condition, but does not indicate definite asthma. Observing the child over time will help make this determination, as asthma will persist and display recurrent symptoms, while a prolonged response to a viral infection will clear.

TABLE 9-1

CAUSES OF WHEEZING

Upper Respiratory Tract	Middle Respiratory Tract	Lower Respiratory Tract
Allergic rhinitis	Tracheomalacia	Asthma
Infectious rhinitis	Tracheoesophageal fistula	Viral bronchiolitis
Adenoidal/tonsillar hypertrophy	Tracheal stenosis	Cystic fibrosis
Foreign body	Bronchial stenosis	Bronchopulmonary dysplasia
Epiglottitis	Vascular ring	Foreign body
Laryngotracheobronchitis	Enlarged lymph nodes	Gastroesophageal reflux with asthma
Vocal cord dysfunction	Tumor	Chronic aspiration
Laryngeal webs	Foreign body	Bronchiectasis
Laryngomalacia	Laryngotracheobronchitis	Tumor

Note: The causes of wheezing have been divided according to the level of the airway obstructed. From a clinical standpoint, upper airway obstruction causes an inspiratory stridor, middle airway obstruction causes inspiratory and expiratory wheezing and lower airway obstruction causes expiratory wheezing.

Laryngotracheomalacia

In this condition, there is softening of the ring cartilage in the trachea and bronchi. It may be the result of viral infections, premature birth or prolonged intubation. The essential features that suggest that this is a cause are the following:

- The infant is not distressed.
- Inspiratory and expiratory wheezing is present. This sign is an indication that the obstruction is in a large central airway.

This condition is not dangerous to the infant, and there is little risk of significant respiratory distress. The parents can be reassured that the infant's wheeze does not indicate a risk of respiratory compromise.

Bronchopulmonary Dysplasia

This condition is a result of premature birth and prolonged assisted ventilation with a high level of inspired O_2. The result of this combination is that there is damage that results in scarring of the lungs with bullous formation and interstitial edema. There is failure to thrive and a prolonged dependence on supplemental O_2.

The key features are the following:

- Extreme prematurity, ventilator, and O_2 dependence
- Scarring, cystic changes, and obstructive lung disease
- These children often have a long-term asthma-like picture

The management is complicated. The essentials are to maintain O_2 and nutrition. These patients will still undergo pulmonary hyperplasia and develop new lung tissue. They also require bronchodilators and are helped by inhaled steroids. The long-term sequela of asthma in BPD is indistinguishable from other forms of asthma, but these children may be refractory to therapy and often have severe symptoms.

Meconium Aspiration

This condition is a problem in infants who have distress at the time of delivery and pass meconium.

The result is that with the first breath, the infant will inhale meconium. It is a cause of serious reactions. The key features are the following:

- Chemical pneumonitis that can be very severe, with pulmonary edema, exudation and transudation of fluid and protein into the alveolar space and the development of a high O_2 requirement. Acutely, these patients may require high O_2 and intensive care therapy. Extracorporeal membrane oxygenation (ECMO) may be needed to provide adequate oxygen levels.
- Long-term sequelae include an asthma-like picture that is usually severe.

Cystic Fibrosis

This condition is one in which there is an abnormal protein at the apex of goblet cells. There is abnormal water and chloride transport leading to thickened mucus and recurrent infections. Infants who have cystic fibrosis have a pleomorphic presentation that can range from subtle to obvious. The usual features are the following:

- Gastrointestinal
  - Meconium ileus
  - Steatorrhea
  - Prolonged jaundice
- Pulmonary
  - Often presents as recurrent wheezing in children under the age of 6 months and this condition is often mistaken for asthma and other chronic respiratory diseases
  - Atelectasis
  - Recurrent pneumonia
  - Chronic cough

Cystic fibrosis is often confused with other diseases. It is reasonable to evaluate a child under the age of 6 months who has persistent wheeze by measuring sweat chloride by sweat iontophoresis.

Cardiac Disease

Chronic and congenital heart disease can be confused with asthma and other causes of obstructive disease in the newborn period.

- Pulmonary venous congestion occurs as part of a number of congenital heart diseases and can present with wheezing. Examples include anomalous pulmonary venous drainage, cor triatriatum and mitral valve stenosis.
- The therapy for this cause of airway obstruction is of the underlying heart disease.

Bronchiolitis

Bronchiolitis is a result of infection with RSV which leads to peribronchial inflammation and floppiness of the airways. The condition can be severe.

The key features are the following:

- Infection by pulmonary inflammatory viruses, especially RSV.
- Mechanical airway obstruction with wheezing on exhalation.
- There is a poor response to bronchodilators because the airways are floppy and bronchodilators reduce the tone of the smooth muscles. This results in increased collapse of the airway and more symptoms.
- The treatment is supportive, and the condition is self-limited.

When Is it Asthma?

Making the distinction between asthma and a prolonged viral response is often very difficult. In many children who have bronchiolitis, there is peribronchial inflammation that is indistinguishable from asthma. These children have repeated episodes of airway obstruction that are similar to asthma.

Several investigators have attempted to define predictors of asthma in children presenting with bronchiolitis. Some criteria that have emerged include the following:

- Children hospitalized with an asthma-like disease under the age of 18 months.
- The presence of allergic manifestations, especially allergic rhinitis.
- A family history of asthma and allergies.
- Exposure to passive cigarette smoke.
- Exposure to nicotine in utero, which Martinez et al. have shown can lead to pulmonary narrowing at birth.
- One of the better correlates with a risk of asthma is elevated specific IgE in response to RSV. Welliver et al. demonstrated that 70% of infants with high titer specific IgE had persistent wheeze and an increased risk of asthma.

Bronchiolitis Versus Asthma

The distinction between asthma and bronchiolitis can be difficult to make acutely. Table 9-2 shows some of the key features that can help to differentiate the two conditions. In bronchiolitis, viruses are the cause of the condition, while viruses are triggers in acute asthma, rather than the cause. Clinically, both conditions appear the same, with

TABLE 9-2

A COMPARISON OF THE ACUTE PRESENTATION OF ASTHMA AND BRONCHIOLITIS

	Bronchiolitis	Asthma
Virus	Cause	Trigger
Appearance	Hyperinflation	Hyperinflation
	Prolonged exhalation	Prolonged exhalation
	Wheeze end expiration	Wheeze midexpiration
Bronchodilator	Poor	Excellent
Steroids	Poor	Excellent
Mechanism	Floppy airway	Inflammation

Note: Essential differences are in the timing of the wheeze, the role of virus, and the response to bronchodilators and steroids.

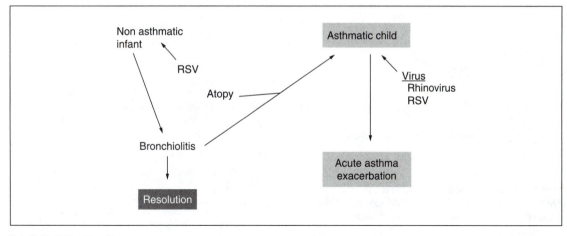

F I G U R E   9 - 2

THE CHANGING ROLE OF VIRUSES IN BRONCHIOLITIS AS OPPOSED TO ASTHMA.

In bronchiolitis, RSV or other inflammatory pulmonary virus causes the condition. The bronchiolitis will resolve in most cases. In the presence of genetic factors and atopy, the infant may develop asthma. Subsequent viral exposure will cause an acute asthmatic episode.

hyperinflation, prolonged exhalation, and wheezing. The timing of the wheeze is later in expiration in bronchiolitis than in asthma and is more musical in nature. This is a difficult distinction to make without a direct comparison. The underlying mechanism is different in the two conditions. In asthma there is swelling and edema of the airways with bronchospasm. In bronchiolitis, the airways are floppy and collapse easily, causing obstruction. For this reason, infants with bronchiolitis do not respond well to bronchodilators, which can cause increase in the floppiness and further collapse. Since inflammation is not a feature of this disease, as opposed to asthma, corticosteroids are also not effective. This comparison is summarized in Table 9-2.

Role of Viruses

Viral infections have a role in initiating the development of asthma. This pathophysiology is discussed in Chap. 3, Hygiene Hypothesis. In infants who are genetically susceptible to develop asthma, exposure to respiratory viruses causes the development of peribronchial inflammation, which probably persists for life. Subsequent exposure to

pulmonary inflammatory viruses causes an acute asthmatic episode, without necessarily causing pneumonia or bronchiolitis. This response is illustrated in Figure 9-2. The role of viral infections in initiating bronchiolitis or triggering an asthmatic episode is dependent on genetic predisposition and other factors. Subsequent exposure in a child who has asthma gives rise to an asthma exacerbation.

The interplay of these genetic and atopic factors is briefly summarized in Figure 9-3. Many factors other than viruses can influence whether a child with a genetic predisposition to asthma develops the disease. These include early exposure to allergens such as animal dander, house dust mites, and mold. There is now consideration of other possibilities, as discussed in the chapter on the Hygiene Hypothesis.

Contribution of IgE to Wheezing in Infants

There is a strong genetic component to the development of asthma. Alleles that contribute to the development of IgE are particularly strong in the association with the development of asthma. These genetic patterns may be the difference between

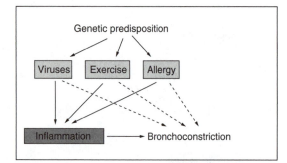

FIGURE   9-3

THE STANDARD MODEL OF ASTHMA IN AN INFANT FOLLOWING VIRAL INFECTION OR OTHER AGENT SUCH AS EARLY ALLERGY EXPOSURE.

The effect of these agents is superimposed on a genetic predisposition, giving rise to long-term peribronchial inflammation. Subsequent bronchoconstriction is then superimposed on this inflammatory base.

patients with bronchiolitis who develop asthma and those who do not. Exposure to allergens early on will increase the risk of developing asthma in these susceptible infants. The outcome has been explored by several investigators. Broadly, of all the infants who develop wheezing under the age of 5 years, 50% will no longer have symptoms after the age of 5–6 years. The remaining children will continue to have asthma symptoms. While it has not been confirmed, it is a reasonable assumption that these are the children who have a genetic predisposition to developing asthma. Children who develop symptoms of wheezing and airway obstruction after the age of 5 years continue to have symptoms and asthma episodes. Martinez et al. have shown that the children who have persistent symptoms after the age of 6 years have atopy and a family history of asthma and allergies. Looked at from another perspective, in children with recurrent wheeze, a history of asthma and the presence of atopy are predictive of life-long symptoms of asthma.

DIAGNOSTIC APPROACH

History

There are several clinical presenting features in infants and children that suggest that the problem

TABLE   9-3

INDICATORS OF POSSIBLE ASTHMA

Cough
With exercise
At night
Recurrent Difficulty Breathing
Recurrent Chest Tightness
Nocturnal Symptoms
Breathlessness
Wheezing
Cough
Associations
Viral infections
Allergen exposure
Vigorous activity
Weather changes
Pollution
Strong emotion

Note: Asthma presents as cough and respiratory distress in infants and children. Symptoms during the night, especially early morning, are typical.

may be asthma, rather that another disease. In asthma, children often present with cough, rather than wheeze. The cough occurs with exercise and activity. The most prominent feature, though, is nocturnal cough. One should be very suspicious of the child who is woken by coughing in the early hours of the morning, often three times or more per week. These findings may be associated with a sensation of chest tightness. Important features are the exposures and activities that trigger the cough. Common associations are listed in Table 9-3. These are triggers that commonly will initiate an acute asthmatic episode. Association of symptoms with trigger events usually associated with asthma strongly suggests that asthma is present.

Other Investigations

Virus Detection

Nasal smears for the detection of RSV, adenovirus, influenza, and parainfluenza can help detect the presence of viral infection. The presence of a virus does not distinguish between asthma and bronchiolitis.

x Ray Chest

Radiography should be used to confirm clinical impressions in wheezing infants. Any child presenting with wheeze for the first time must have an x ray of the chest. The radiographic appearance is typical in many of the conditions in the differential of the wheezing child as noted above. For example, a foreign body in a bronchus may produce hyperinflation of one lung; cystic fibrosis can present with subsegmental atelectasis of the upper lobes and volume loss; there may be cardiomegaly in heart disease.

On the other hand, a chest x ray is not necessary for every episode in a diagnosed asthmatic. The radiograph should be obtained only if there is a specific question to be answered. An example would be the child who suddenly deteriorates and the x ray is needed to exclude a pneumothorax. Another example is the child who has asthma and present with localizing pulmonary findings and fever where an x ray will confirm or disprove pneumonia.

Sweat Chloride

Where cystic fibrosis is suspected, a properly performed sweat chloride is diagnostic or excludes the diagnosis. The test should be performed in a center where it is used frequently, as in a Cystic Fibrosis Center.

Specialized Radiologic Studies

These specialized tests should be used for specific indications.

Esophagram

This study is useful in detecting the presence of compression of the esophagus as would be found in vascular abnormalities. It is also useful in finding abnormalities of swallowing. Tracheoesophageal fistulas can be subtle, especially if they are of the "H" type and a careful esophagram will detect the defect.

CT scan and MRI

CAT scan or MRI of the chest should be used to resolve a diagnostic dilemma. An example would be to detect a peribronchial mass or to confirm a vascular anomaly.

Further Studies

Further specialize work up depends on the presentation and should be applied as indicated.

- Cardiac studies
- Immune workup (see Chap. 13)

THERAPY

The treatment of the wheezing infant is essentially that of the underlying disease. Surgical correction is indicated for cardiac defects, esophageal fistulae and vascular rings and slings compressing the bronchi or trachea.

Role of Bronchodilators

The use of a bronchodilator as a trial of therapy can distinguish asthma from bronchiolitis. While not infallible, asthma will respond to albuterol, while bronchiolitis will not. This bedside test may be helpful to make a preliminary distinction.

Role of Steroids

Steroids have little effect in viral illnesses, and should be reserved for inflammatory conditions.

CONCLUSION

The etiology of wheezing in infants is complex, and a careful history and physical examination is needed to distinguish the cause. Specific tests should be used, and therapy is essentially the care of the underlying condition. It should be remembered that the wheeze is only a symptom, not the disease.

Suggested Reading

Balfour-Lynn, I. M. (2003). Asthma in cystic fibrosis. *J R Soc Med* **96**(Suppl. 43): 30–4.

Bancalari, E., N. Claure, et al. (2003). Bronchopulmonary dysplasia: changes in pathogenesis, epidemiology and definition. *Semin Neonatol* **8**(1): 63–71.

Cleary, G. M. and T. E. Wiswell (1998). Meconium-stained amniotic fluid and the meconium aspiration syndrome. An update. *Pediatr Clin North Am* **45**(3): 511–29.

Faubion, W. A., Jr. and N. N. Zein (1998). Gastroesophageal reflux in infants and children. *Mayo Clin Proc* **73**(2): 166–73.

Klingner, M. C. and J. Kruse (1999). Meconium aspiration syndrome: pathophysiology and prevention. *J Am Board Fam Pract* **12**(6): 450–66.

Orenstein, S. R. (2001). An overview of reflux-associated disorders in infants: apnea, laryngospasm, and aspiration. *Am J Med* **111**(Suppl. 8A): 60S–63S.

Sarani, B., M. Gleiber, et al. (2002). Esophageal pH monitoring, indications, and methods. *J Clin Gastroenterol* **34**(3): 200–6.

Vaucher, Y. E. (2002). Bronchopulmonary dysplasia: an enduring challenge. *Pediatr Rev* **23**(10): 349–58.

Wagener, J. S., M. K. Sontag, et al. (2003). Newborn screening for cystic fibrosis. *Curr Opin Pediatr* **15**(3): 309–15.

Wang, L. and S. D. Freedman (2002). Laboratory tests for the diagnosis of cystic fibrosis. *Am J Clin Pathol* **117**(Suppl.): S109–15.

10

RECURRENT INFECTIONS AND IMMUNE DEFECTS

RECURRENT INFECTIONS

Recurrent or persistent infections are common occurrences. The key clinical indication of an immunologic abnormality is a pattern of repeated or persistent infections. These infections are likely to occur at multiple, rather than a single site.

Site

The usual site of repeated infections is in a hollow viscus; sinus cavities, middle ear, lungs, and gastrointestinal tract. Although the urinary tract is a hollow organ, it is self-flushing, so recurrent urinary tract infections are most frequently due to mechanical causes such as vesicoureteric reflux, rather than an immune defect.

General Approach

The cause of recurrent infections lies either with the organism or with the host.

Organism

An inadequate choice of antibiotic is the most usual reason for persistent infections. Very commonly, the organism is resistant or inadequately treated (Table 10-1).

Resistant. Increasingly, organisms have become resistant to commonly used antibiotics. This problem could give the impression of an immune defect.

Sequestrated. Bacteria may be isolated in an area that has a poor blood supply, is surrounded by necrotic tissue or is cystic in type. An example is a sequestration of a portion of the lung, usually the lower lobe. In this situation, the lobe has tenuous connections to the bronchi, and is only supplied by the bronchial blood vessels. This area does not provide gas exchange, and is prone to repeated infections because of poor drainage. Another common sequestered site is bone.

Unusual or unexpected. An organism that is not usually the cause of infection at the site, such as *Pseudomonas* sp. otitis media, can cause confusion and a poor response to antibiotics.

Antibiotic errors. This is probably the most frequent cause of persistent and recurrent infections.

TABLE 10-1
CAUSES OF RECURRENT INFECTION

Organism
  Resistant
  Sequestrated
  Unusual or unexpected
  Antibiotic errors
    Wrong drug
    Wrong dose
    Incomplete course

Host
  Local causes—obstruction
    In the lumen
    In the wall
    Outside the wall
  Systemic
    Immune defects
    Cardiac defects
    Cystic fibrosis

Note: The causes of recurrent infection lie either with the organism or with the host. The local causes usually relate to obstruction of a hollow viscus.

- Wrong drug
- Wrong dose
- Incomplete course

Host

The underlying mechanism is obstruction to the lumen and distal stasis with subsequent bacterial overgrowth.

Local causes

- In the lumen

In children, a foreign body is a likely cause. In adults this is more often a problem among those who are impaired (such as in drug and alcohol consumption).

- In the wall

The usual cause is a benign or malignant mass

- Outside the wall

There may be compression of the bronchus from outside by a benign or malignant mass, or a vascular anomaly such as a vascular ring or sling.

Systemic

- Immune defects
- Cardiac defects
- Cystic fibrosis

INVESTIGATION OF RECURRENT INFECTIONS

History

There are several questions that can help delineate the cause of recurrent infections.

- Site of infection
  - Same site

Infections that occur in the same anatomic site imply a mechanical process causing obstruction with stasis distal to the obstructed site leading to bacterial overgrowth. Otitis media and sinusitis are common examples of mechanical mechanisms.

  - Multiple sites

The implication in this scenario is that there is a systemic defect, especially if the sites are involved at different times.
Exception: Urinary tract
Infections in this site imply a mechanical problem, as the urinary tract is a self-flushing system. Repeated urinary tract infections indicate a mechanical problem, such a vesicoureteric reflux.

- Is the infection bacterial?

Bacterial infection is suggestive of a defect in immunoglobulin production. This is a more common form of immune defect than T-cell/macrophage axis problems, which present with viral infections as well as bacterial.

- Does it clear completely?

This question distinguishes persistent from recurrent infections. Persistent infections are more likely to be caused by a problem with the organism, such as being resistant to antibiotics.

  - Travel history

There is always the potential for an unexpected organism when patients travel to foreign countries that have poor hygiene or are more tropical.

• Family history

There is a strong familial and genetic pattern in congenital immune defects. The family history may reveal siblings or other family members who had recurrent infections or even died at a very young age of infections.

• Associated abnormalities

Many congenital immune defects are associated with developmental abnormalities. A typical example is the Di George syndrome, where thymic defects are associated with facial abnormalities, aortic defects, and absence of the parathyroid gland. Immune dysfunction is often seen as part of specific syndromes, such as Ataxia Telangiectasia (AT) and Wiskott-Aldrich syndrome.

Laboratory

x ray
Sweat chloride
Immune studies

DEFECTS OF IMMUNE FUNCTION

The principles of immune function and development of the immune system are presented in Chap. 1. Defects of immune function are essentially errors in development or a breakdown in normal cell action or intercell communication.

Suspicion of Immune Defects

The final common pathway in a systemic pattern of recurrent infections is an immune defect or blockade. A systemic defect is suggested by

• Multiple sites involved at different times
• Recurrent rather than persistent infections; the patient will appear to be normal between episodes
• Bacterial infections are more likely as an indicator of underlying immune defect
• There may be a family history of immune defect or recurrent infections

• Other defects are often present, especially congenital abnormalities
• Onset may be at any age, but is more usual among infants and young children

Clinical Presentation

Some clinical scenarios might indicate the following syndromes:

• *Bruton's agammaglobulinemia*: An 8-month-old male infant who has had five episodes of otitis media and one episode of pneumonia. Growth rate is delayed.
• *Common variable immune defect*: A 6-year-old who was previously well now has had four episodes of otitis media and pneumonia in the past year. She has also had two episodes of sinusitis and pneumonia.
• *Di George syndrome*: A 6-week-old male has persistent hypocalcemia, cardiac defects that include an interrupted aortic arch and had two episodes of bacterial sepsis.
• *Pan hypogammaglobulinemia secondary to lymphoma*: A 20-year-old female presents with recent onset of recurrent sinusitis, pneumonia, and otitis media. There are enlarged cervical and supraclavicular nodes present. She has previously been well.
• *Hypogammaglobulinemia and complement deficiency*: A young adult male in boot camp in the Marines presents with classical symptoms and signs of acute meningitis. Spinal puncture reveals large numbers of meningococci with very few polymorphonuclear cells. CSF protein is elevated.

DEFECTS IN IMMUNE FUNCTION

General Principles

Clinical Features

Recurrent infections are the key feature of an immune defect. There are often distinct patterns of infection that suggest the possibility of disordered immune function. These patterns are discussed below. There is a correlation between the type of immune defect and the pattern of symptoms and signs.

Several broad groups of symptoms raise the suspicion of an immune defect:

- Pathogenic bacterial infections, often upper and lower airway infections, sepsis, and meningitis.
- Opportunistic infections by organism that are not usually pathogenic or invasive in healthy hosts. Examples would include the following:
  - *Mycoplasma pneumoniae.*
  - *Pneumocystis carinii.*
  - Atypical mycobacteria.
- Viral infections—overwhelming, rather than recurrent.
- Patients with T-cell defects may have viral sepsis and disseminated infections with viruses that are usually localized, such as herpes simplex infections.

Recurrent infections tend to occur in hollow viscera, e.g., the middle ear, lung, and bowel. The urinary tract is an exception. While the ureters are hollow organs, and the kidneys are a site for recurrent infections, these are seldom associated with immune deficiency. Generally, recurrent urinary tract infections are caused by mechanical problems, such as ureteric reflux.

Presentations of Immune Defects

In broad terms, the way in which recurrent infections present can indicate where the underlying defect of immune function might be (Table 10-2).

B-Cell Defects

For patients who present with recurrent bacterial sinusitis, otitis media, pneumonia, meningitis or sepsis, a defect in B-cell function should be considered. The tonsils and adenoids are rich in B cells and provide a first line barrier against infection. Thus, the organisms that occur in B-cell deficits are the predominant cause of respiratory infection;

TABLE 10-2

INFECTION PATTERN FOR DIFFERENT CELL DEFECTS

Defect	Types of Organisms	Types of Infections
B cells	Recurrent/persistent bacterial	Otitis media
		Pneumonia
		Meningitis
		Septicemia
T cells	Recurrent/unusual/ opportunistic	Sepsis
	Viral/bacterial	Pneumocystis
		Mycoplasma
		Atypical Mycobacteria
		Interstitial pneumonitis
		Unusual infections
		Overwhelming infections
Polymorphonuclear cells	Bacterial	Cold abscess
		Sepsis
		Fungal sepsis
Complement	Bacterial	Meningitis
		Abscess
		Sepsis

Note: The pattern of recurrent infections reflects the possible immune defect.

TABLE 10-3

PATTERNS OF IGA DEFICIENCY AND THE PROBABILITY THAT EACH PATTERN WOULD LEAD TO INFECTION

Serum IgA	Secretory IgA	Frequency	Cause Infections
Absent	Present	Common	Rarely
Absent	Absent	Less common	Yes
Present	Absent	Rare	Yes

Pneumococcus, Haemophilus, Staphylococcus and *Moraxella* species. The consequence of B-cell dysfunction is a defect in antibody production. From a pathophysiologic perspective, abnormalities in B-cell development can occur at any point along the normal embryogenic pathway (see Chap. 1). These defects include absence of mature B cells, the presence of T cells that suppress B-cell function, an inability of B cells to transform into plasma cells or of plasma cells to secrete immunoglobulins.

Antibody Defects

Defects of antibody production can be partial, involving only one class or subclass of immunoglobulin or involve all major classes (IgG, IgM, and IgA) in pan-hypogammaglobulinemia.

Partial

IgA deficiency. Low to absent serum IgA is the most common serum immunoglobulin defect with a general pediatric frequency of 1 in 600. The majority of these children do not exhibit evidence of immune defect, and this finding is of questionable clinical significance. IgA functions predominantly as a secretory antibody, and absence of this form is more likely to have an association with infections. There are three patterns of IgA deficiency as shown in Table 10-3.

While more difficult to establish, the absence of secretory IgA is more likely to have an association with infections of sinuses, middle ear, and GI tract than a lack of serum antibody with secretory antibody present.

Low or absent IgG2 levels in serum have been found in children with IgA deficiency. These patients tend to be susceptible to recurrent infections with *Haemophilus* and *Pneumococcus* species. These children will usually fail to make antibodies in response to *Haemophilus influenzae* immunization.

IgG subclasses. There are four subclasses of IgG (Table 10-4).

TABLE 10-4

SUBCLASSES 1–4 OF IGG ARE SHOWN WITH THEIR PRESUMED ANTIBACTERIAL FUNCTION

Class	Percent of Total	Function
G1	80	General bacterial
G2	12	Encapsulated organisms
G3	5	General
G4	2	Possible reaginic effect

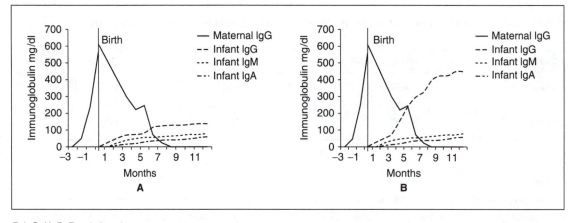

FIGURE 10-1

IMMUNOGLOBULIN PATTERN IN A NEWBORN.

Immunoglobulin pattern in a newborn with transient hypogammaglobulinemia is shown in graph **A** on the left. IgG does rise slowly after birth, while transplacentally acquired maternal IgG declines. IgM and IgA are normal. For comparison, the normal postnatal pattern is presented in graph **B** on the right, showing the normal IgG curve.

The majority of IgG falls into the G1 class. IgG3 and IgG4 constitute a small fraction of the total immunoglobulin, and the contribution to the immune response by these immunoglobulins is unclear. There is evidence to suggest that IgG4 may be involved in allergic (reaginic) type reactions, but this concept is controversial. IgG2 appears to prevent infection with organisms that have a polysaccharide capsule, namely *Haemophilus* and *Pneumococcus* species.

For this reason, the clearest association of an IgG subclass immune defect is that of IgG2 deficiency which has been linked to recurrent rhinosinusitus and otitis media due to *Haemophilus* or pneumococcal infection.

Transient hypogammaglobulinemia of infancy. This is a benign condition in which there is a delay in switching from production of IgM to IgG during the first 15–18 months of life. The cause for this delay is not known.

The infant typically presents with upper airway infections and usually does not have major or life-threatening infections. Growth and development are usually normal. Lymphadenopathy is unusual, and tonsillar tissue is normal.

Serum immunoglobulin measurements have a typical pattern. There are normal IgM and IgA levels with low to low normal IgG. Immunization will result in a normal antibody response (Figure 10-1).

Generally, these children produce IgG normally by 18 months.

This condition is probably not clinically significant, and does not normally require replacement gamma-globulin therapy.

Pan Hypogammaglobulinemia

In this group of conditions, serum IgG, IgA, and IgM are all at low levels or absent. These children tend to have serious infections, especially of the respiratory tract and upper airway. Pneumonia is common, and over time, these patients often develop saccular bronchiectasis, often despite regular therapy.

Bruton's agammaglobulinemia. These children tend to present from 4 to 6 months of age. This is an X-linked recessive condition, in which the defect has been traced to the gene locus that encodes for B-cell tyrosine kinase. The condition occurs with a frequency of 1/75,000 live births. This enzyme is necessary for the maturation of B cells. In its absence, B cells do not mature beyond the precursor stage. The resultant cells are not capable of developing into plasma cells or synthesizing antibody. These patients therefore have very low levels of IgG, IgM, and IgA in plasma. They are prone to infections with bacteria, often respiratory pathogens.

Physical findings include. Recurrent bacterial infections involve sinuses, middle ear, lung, and often have systemic spread.

Lymphoid tissue is often absent, and tonsils are not visible, despite repeated upper airway infections. A finding of pus that contains many organisms but few polymorphonuclear cells is particularly suggestive of an opsonic defect of immunoglobulin or complement.

Common variable immune deficiency diseases (CVID). This group of conditions encompasses a wide variety of underlying defects in B-cell function. These include cells that suppress B-cell function, inability of B cells to transform into plasma cells, and lack of glycosylation of immunoglobulin.

The onset ranges from the first year into adulthood. When the onset is in adulthood, there is a concern that the patient may have an underlying lymphoid malignancy.

Like Bruton's, these patients present with recurrent infections, usually of the upper airway involving sinuses and middle ear.

Often, lymphadenopathy is present. Many of the underlying defects in B-cell function involve inadequate feedback mechanisms. As a result, B cells continue to proliferate. Even though immunoglobulin is being produced, there is a breakdown of specific feedback shut-off mechanisms. Tonsillar tissue may be present or absent.

Many patients present with arthralgia or even arthritis. Patients who are on replacement gamma globulins may notice arthralgia before the dose is due.

Hyper IgE syndrome (Buckley syndrome). This is an unusual condition that has an equal sex incidence and is inherited as an autosomal recessive. These children present with recurrent abscesses that involve skin and viscera. Visceral abscesses can be pulmonary, hepatic, renal, perianal, or occur within sinus cavities. Because of the recurrent skin infections, these patients all develop coarse facial features. The most usual organism is *Staphylococcus*, but patients are infected by other bacteria and fungi.

The use of matched bone marrow has been curative.

Cellular Defects

Note: With a few exceptions, B cells function poorly in humans in the absence of T cells. Thus, nonfunctioning or poorly functioning T cells result in secondary antibody deficiency or the production of immunoglobulin that does not bind specifically to antigen and does not have antibody function.

Clinical Presentation

Congenital defects of T cells present early in life. These infants are usually ill with a combination of susceptibility to severe infections and congenital abnormalities. T-cell defects are often part of recognized congenital syndromes.

The characteristics of T-cell defects are shown in Table 10-5.

There is usually an early onset of infection, within the first 6 months to a year. The organisms that are involved are often not pathogens in normal individuals. *Pneumocystis carinii* pneumonia is regarded as pathognomonic of poorly or nonfunctional T cells, as is pneumonia caused by cytomegalovirus outside of the immediate newborn period. These pulmonary infections are often interstitial in nature. Other organisms that cause problems are normally weak pathogens, such as Klebsiella and *Pseudomonas* species. Opportunistic organism, like atypical mycobacteria also seldom occur in individuals with normally functional T cells. Many of the forms of congenital T-cell defects are associated with congenital anomalies that draw attention to the condition early. These infants and young children are often very ill, and are easily overwhelmed by infection, especially sepsis.

The range of T-cell defects is shown in Table 10-6. They can be considered in two broad categories; T-cell defects with normal B-cell function, and the combination of both T-cell and B-cell defects.

TABLE 10-5

TYPICAL PATTERNS OF INFECTION THAT ARE FOUND IN PATIENTS WHO LACK FUNCTIONAL T CELLS

Defect	Types of Organisms	Types of Infections
T Cells	Recurrent	Sepsis
	Unusual	Pneumocystis
	Opportunistic	Mycoplasma
	Viral	Atypical mycobacteria
	Bacterial	Interstitial pneumonitis
		Unusual infections
		Overwhelming infections

With Normal B Cells

Di George syndrome. This syndrome is a triad of immune defect with absent T cells, aortic arch defects, and hypoparathyroidism presenting with persistent hypocalcemia. The underlying defect belongs to the broader family of chromosomal defects based on deletions on chromosome 22q11—the 22q11.2 region is linked to Di George syndrome. There are characteristic facial features with a short philtrum of the upper lip, hypertelorism, an antimongoloid slant to the eyes, mandibular hypoplasia, and rounded, low-set, often notched ears. Hand abnormalities may also be seen. Cardiac defects include anomalies of the

TABLE 10-6

T-CELL DEFECTS CAN OCCUR WITH B-CELL DEFICIENCIES OR ALONE. THE SYNDROMES THAT ARE ASSOCIATED WITH EACH GROUP ARE PRESENTED IN THIS TABLE

T-cell Defect	Type	Signs
With normal B cells	Di George syndrome (chromosome 22q11 family)	Absence of mature T cells
		Severe infections
	Developmental abnormalities	Interrupted aortic arch
		Hypoparathyroidism with hypocalcemia
		Severe viral and bacterial infections
With reduced B cells	Severe combined immunodeficiency	Severe viral
	Subtypes:	Severe bacterial
	ADA deficiency	Opportunistic infections
	Jak3 deficiency	Unusual organisms
	RAG deficiency	
	PNP deficiency	

great vessels (right-sided aortic arch, interrupted aortic arch, truncus arteriosus, and atrial and ventricular septal defects). Esophageal atresia and bifid uvula may also occur.

The immune defects result from absence of the thymus during the critical period of early embryogenesis. The result is the complete absence of mature T cells, and severe immune deficiency. Despite the risk of overwhelming infections, the infants more usually are detected because of persistent hypocalcemia or cardiac defect.

Therapy consists of bone marrow transplantation. Grafting with thymic epithelium has had some success with restoration of T cells, but there is a very high risk of development of lymphoma.

The broad categorization of complex T-cell defects is shown in Table 10-6. These are rare conditions where T cells and B cells are absent. The absence of functional T cells and B cells results is susceptibility to viruses, bacteria, and organism that are not usually pathogens.

With Abnormal B Cells

Wiskott-Aldrich. This is an X-linked (mapped to Xp11.22-11.23) condition that is a triad of symptoms. This locus codes for the Wiskott-Aldrich Syndrome Protein that blocks GTPase. There is a mix of immunoglobulin defects and T-cell deficiencies. These patients have extensive eczema, thrombocytopenia with characteristically small platelets, and an immune defect that has a characteristic pattern in immuno-globulin; IgG is normal, IgM is very low, and IgA and IgE are elevated. Synthesis and catabolism of immunoglobulins are accelerated. These patients have features of immunoglobulin defects with infection predominantly by encapsulated organisms from an early age. They develop T-cell defects later as there is progressive loss of T-cell function and numeric decrease. Antibody titers to protein antigens fall over time, and anamnestic responses deteriorate.

Severe combined immunodeficiency diseases (SCID). There are several forms of this type of rare immune defect. In common to all types, there is a defect of T cells and B cells resulting in a profound loss of immune function. The most frequent form is X-linked (42% of cases). Onset of symptoms is within the first 2–3 months after birth. Infants usually have frequent episodes of diarrhea, pneumonia, otitis, sepsis, and cutaneous infections. Despite initially normal growth, there is marked failure to thrive. Persistent infections with opportunistic organisms and usually weak pathogens such as *Candida albicans, Pneumocystis carinii* and varicella-zoster virus can lead to early death, as is typically seen in severe T-cell deficiency.

The most striking defect is that these infants are profoundly lymphopenic. On immune workup, there is an absence of lymphocyte-proliferative responses to mitogens, antigens, and allogeneic cells in vitro. Cord blood lymphocyte count lower than 4000/mm^3 should be regarded as lymphopenic. Serum immunoglobulin concentrations are profoundly depressed, and there is no response to immunization. Paradoxically, despite the severe lack of lymphocytes, there may be elevation of non-immunoglobulin producing B cells. These B cells are poorly functional, and do not recover even after successful marrow transplantation. These patients also demonstrate poor thymic development. There is absence of splenic and tonsillar lymphoid structures, including germinal centers. One defined defect is the inability to produce a gamma$_c$ chain common to cytokines.

Because they lack competent immune cells, these infants are at risk for graft-versus-host disease (GVHD). GVHD is a condition in which competent immune cells placed into an immunodeficient host reject the immunodeficient host, ultimately destroying it. It is an ever present problem in bone marrow transplantation. It can also result from maternal T cells that cross into the fetal circulation while the SCID infant is in utero. More conventionally, it can also result from T lymphocytes infused into the infant with nonirradiated blood products or even when performing allogeneic bone marrow transplant.

Adenosine deaminase deficiency. This defect accounts for approximately 15% of patients with

SCID. Milder forms of the disease that present in adulthood have been reported. The defect lies on chromosome 20q13-ter, and results in the accumulation of adenosine, 2′-deoxyadenosine, and 2′-O-methyladenosine in rapidly dividing cells, like T cells. These metabolites trigger programmed cell death (apoptosis) when they build up in cells. These patients present similarly to all SCID patients, with severe and opportunistic infections of viral and bacterial origins. In addition, there are characteristic rachitic rosary-like rib-cage abnormalities with chondrodysplasia. This condition is characterized by profound lymphopenia, without elevated B cell as is seen in other forms of SCID. There may be normal natural killer (NK) cell function. They have evidence of thymic arrest, rather than absence on the thymus.

Specific treatment for ADA. Matched T-cell-depleted bone marrow transplantation is the treatment of choice. In this disease, where there is a defined enzyme defect, attempts have been made to replace the adenosine deaminase. Polyethylene glycol-modified bovine ADA (PEG-ADA has been administered by weekly subcutaneous injection with clinical and immunologic improvement. PEG-ADA therapy is not as efficient as marrow transplant, and should be considered if transplant is not feasible. Gene therapy has been attempted, but has met with little success.

Janus Kinase 3 deficiency. This defect is clinically a variant of X-linked SCID. Patients present in an identical manner with the same range of infections. Unlike ADA defect, B cells are elevated while T cell and NK cells are absent. Like the X-linked form, there is an inability to produce a common gamma$_c$ chain. In fact, Jak3 is the molecule associated with this gamma$_c$ chain.

Recombinase-activating gene (RAG-1 or RAG-2) deficiencies. While infants with RAG-1 and RAG-2 deficiencies are clinically indistinguishable from other patients with SCID, they have a distinct lymphocyte profile. These patients lack both T cells and B cells. Their primary circulating lymphocytes are NK cells. In lacking the RAG enzymes, these lymphocytes have a functional

inability to form antigen receptors through genetic recombination.

Purine nucleoside phosphorylase deficiency (PNP). This is a rare condition, with only 40 patients found to have PNP deficiency. They have low but not absent T-cell function, and usually present later than patients with SCID. Presenting infections are generalized vaccinia or varicella infections, lymphosarcoma, and graft-versus-host type disease from blood transfusion. A high percentage of patients have neurologic abnormalities or autoimmune diseases. There is profound T-cell lymphopenia, but immunoglobulins are high. The gene defect lies in the 14q13.1 region.

Chronic mucocutaneous candidiasis (CMCC). This unusual condition may be a clinical example of immune tolerance. It is a collection of immune deficiency syndromes characterized by persistent or recurrent Candida infections of the skin, nails, and mucous membranes. The onset is usually during the first 3–5 years of life. Autoimmune endocrinopathy commonly accompanies the condition. This takes the form of hypoparathyroidism (70% of patients) Addison's disease (37%). Hypothyroidism, diabetes, and pernicious anemia have also been described. Oral mucous membranes are most affected. Skin and nail lesions may be sharply demarcated scaly erythematous macular rash or, more unusually, granulomatous. The lesions remain superficial and do not become systemic. Esophageal involvement may cause dysphagia.

Immune changes in CMCC. Characteristically, delayed skin reactivity to Candida is absent. Isolated lymphocytes do not proliferate in response to Candida antigen in vitro. Antibody production to a number of antigens, including *Candida,* is normal. Most patients have a selective cellular defect against *Candida,* whereas others may have a more variable T-cell immune deficiency. Plasma factors that inhibit lymphocyte-proliferative responses to *Candida* antigen have also been described. Curiously, this inhibitory activity resolves with treatment of the candidal infection and return of positive delayed skin reactivity and in vitro proliferative response to

Candida. Antigen-specific suppressor T cells have also been reported.

Treatment of CMCC. Systemic antifungal therapy with such oral agents as ketoconazole, fluconazole, itraconazole, or parenteral amphotericin B is needed to control this condition. Antifungal therapy must be accompanied by immunologic reconstitution. Immunologic improvement may be achieved using transfer factor. A combination of transfer factor and fetal thymus transplantation has been successful.

Very Rare Conditions

- Zeta chain-associated protein (zap-70) deficiency—results in CD8 depletion
- Inability to express the T-cell receptor-CD3 complex—severe T-cell deficiency
- Abnormal interferon gamma receptor-1—inability to control mycobacteria
- MHC class II deficiency—present as a milder variant of SCID with severe diarrhea
- Leukocyte adhesion molecule deficiencies

DEFECTS IN POLYMORPHONUCLEAR CELLS

There are two forms of PMN deficiency, numeric and functional.

Numeric Defects

In general, defects in the number of PMNs results in sepsis first with seeding of organisms to cause chronic infections at multiple site especially bone.

Numeric defects are the most frequent, and result from neutropenia of any cause. Most of the causes are due to decreased granulocyte production which occurs as a result of a reaction to drugs, infections, or neoplastic conditions. In some patients, the cause remains obscure.

Cyclic Neutropenia

Cyclic neutropenia is a condition that is characterized by profound decrease in circulating neutrophils, often as low as $50/mm^3$. The condition has a periodicity of about 21 days, with a wide range in time interval. There is a maturational arrest in the myeloid line during the neutropenic periods. The diagnosis is made by taking daily blood counts over a 4–6-week period.

There may be increased destruction, as is seen in autoimmune disorders, such as lupus erythematosus.

Congenital Neutropenias

Congenital neutropenia is predominantly an autosomal recessive condition, but autosomal dominant forms have been described. Patients present with severe bacterial infections in early infancy.

The Shwachman syndrome consists of neutropenia with pancreatic insufficiency. These patients have recurrent infections with growth failure and steatorrhea in early childhood.

Functional Defects

Where PMNs are unable to kill organisms, but do not have problems with phagocytosis, patients develop a *"cold" abscess*. In this lesion, there is an inability to kill the organism, but PMNs ingest it thus confining it to a site. It continues to multiply in the PMN, causing significant destruction of tissue. Since PMNs are not activated, there is no release of inflammatory mediators. While there may be extensive local tissue destruction, there are no local reactions typical of abscess formation: heat, redness, and pain. Organisms that are usually causative for these lesions are catalase positive. Common examples are *Staphylococcus aureus*, *Pseudomonas* and *Serratia* species. *Pneumococcus* and *Haemophilus* are catalase negative and are not causes of infection.

Chronic granulomatous disease. This is the most frequent of disorders that involve the respiratory burst pathway, but is still rare at about 1/500,000 live births. The defect lies in the pentose phosphate shunt pathway of phagocytic cells, specifically in conversion of NADP to NADPH, during which H_2O_2 is produced with NADPH oxidase. H_2O_2 is important in killing ingested bacteria. NADPH interacts with four components of cytochrome b245 any of which may be low or abnormal in

CGD: gp91phox (57%, X-linked), p47phox (33%, recessive), p33phox (5%, recessive) and p67phox (5%, recessive) (phox: phagocyte oxidase). The result of these defects is defective intracellular killing of bacterial and fungal organisms that produce catalase, and thus remove H_2O_2 produced by the bacteria.

Cold abscess formation is characteristic and considerable tissue damage may occur. Lesions are found in the skin, lymph nodes, liver, lungs, or other viscera. Osteomyelitis may be caused by bacteria and fungi such as Aspergillus. The age of onset of CGD is usually in infancy, but may be later. Chronic, partly controlled infections lead to the characteristic granulomas in GUT, liver, urinary tract, lung, skin, and other viscera.

Blood counts reveal normal neutrophil numbers. These cells have reduced superoxide ion (O_2^-) production in response to phagocytosis or stimulation artificially with phorbol myristate acetate (PMA). Measured chemotactic adherence, and phagocytic functions of these cells are normal. The diagnosis of CGD is made when one can demonstrate an inability of neutrophils from the patient to undergo a respiratory burst after phagocytosis or PMA stimulation, that is, to generate superoxide ions. One measurement tool employs nitroblue tetrazolium (NBT) which is relatively insensitive. Definitive diagnosis involves demonstrating lack of gp91phox or p47phox.

Treatment

Antibiotics: Cephalosporins, trimethoprim-sulfamethoxazole, and aminoglycosides are useful in controlling infections. There is always a risk of developing resistance to beta lactam antibiotics, but drugs such as Vancomycin should be reserved for specific indications such as methicillin resistant organisms. Many patients die from fungal infections, which are difficult to manage and are resistant to therapy.

Combination therapy: Amphotericin B has been used in combination with granulocyte infusions with some success in clearing the infection. The addition of IFN-gamma subcutaneously three times a week has also proved efficacious.

Transplant: HLA identical marrow transplantation is the only curative procedure. It should be performed as early in the course of the disease as possible.

Ataxia Telangiectasia

Ataxia telangiectasia (AT) is an autosomal recessive condition that belongs to the group of neurocutaneous syndromes. This disease group includes neurofibromatosis and tuberous sclerosis. The key clinical feature is progressive cerebellar ataxia with prominent oculocutaneous telangiectasias. Immune deficiency is manifest in chronic sinopulmonary disease with other infections and a high incidence of malignancy because of increased susceptibility of the chromosomes to damage and resultant breaks, especially on chromosomes 7 and 14.

Immunologic defects in Ataxia Telangiectasia. The most obvious immune defect is selective IgA deficiency, found in 50–80%, and an abnormal IgM that is of low molecular weight. Total IgG, and especially IgG2, may be decreased. There is loss of the delayed skin test (T-cell mediated) and prolonged graft survival. In vitro tests of lymphocyte function have generally shown moderately depressed proliferative responses. The thymus is hypoplastic, exhibits poor organization, and is lacking in Hassall's corpuscles.

Chediak-Higashi Syndrome

This is a rare autosomal recessive syndrome that is characterized by oculocutaneous albinism and susceptibility to recurrent infections, especially of the respiratory tract. The disease is characterized by giant lysosomal granules in the cells of most organs, but especially in neutrophils. Poor functioning of the neutrophils is caused by these abnormal lysosomes that are unable to fuse with phagosomes and lyse ingested bacteria. Cytotoxic T lymphocytes and NK cells are absent. Eighty-five percent of patients enter an accelerated phase, characterized by fever, jaundice, hepatosplenomegaly, lymphadenopathy, pancytopenia, bleeding diathesis, and neurologic changes. This condition is usually fatal. The only therapy is HLA compatible bone marrow transplantation.

CLINICAL MANIFESTATIONS OF COMPLEMENT DEFICIENCIES

Complement Defect	Disease Pattern
C1 esterase inhibitor	Hereditary angioedema
C1, C2, C3, C4, C8, C9	Rheumatoid diseases
C3, C5, C6, C8, C9	Recurrent infections

Note: Clinical manifestations of complement defects fall into categories depending on the components that are missing.

COMPLEMENT DEFECTS

Primary complement defects that are associated with immune defects are relatively rare conditions.

The clinical manifestations of complement deficiencies are shown in Table 10-7.

Defects in C3 and C5 are predominantly associated with bacterial infections including *Pneumococcus* and *Haemophilus*, but other infections such as *Neisseria*, can also occur.

Defects in the late complement components, such as C6 and C8 are particularly associated with infections with *Neisseria meningitidis* and gonorrhea. Systemic infections and repeated infections with these organisms should arouse suspicion of a possible complement defect.

SECONDARY IMMUNE DEFECTS

AIDS

The acquired immunodeficiency syndrome was described in 1981 when the Centers for Disease Control (CDC) noted a high frequency of reported males with cytomegalovirus pneumonia (CMV). Outside of the newborn period, CMV pneumonia is highly indicative of T-cell deficiency. A retrovirus, the human immunodeficiency virus (HIV), is the cause of this syndrome. The virus is transmitted predominantly by sexual contact, especially male homosexual contact. Blood transmission has also been reported, and the screening of blood bank products has been a very important measure in controlling spread of the disease. It is now recognized that there may be a prolonged dormancy period, and progression of the disease may be slow. This is partly due to the fact that there is earlier diagnosis and awareness of the disease and patients are detected before they have severe pulmonary infections.

Prevalence

From the onset AIDS to 2001, nearly 60 million people worldwide have been infected with the virus, and an estimated 40 million people live with HIV. The worst area in the world is sub-Saharan Africa where over 28 million people in the region currently live with HIV, a prevalence of 8%. The region is the only one where more women than men are infected by the virus. Without the problem of AIDS, the predicted life expectancy in sub-Saharan Africa would be 62 years; it currently stands at 47 years. AIDS killed 2.3 million people in 2001 and there were 3.4 million new HIV infections.

The fastest rate of increase is in Eastern Europe and Russia with a 15-fold rise in infections from 1999 to 2001. Injected drug use is the main culprit. China had a 67% rise in 2001 and India has also experienced a rapid rise of the disease.

In two counties where the disease was rife, Cambodia and Thailand, large scale prevention programs are showing some success.

Immunology

HIV is a retrovirus (an RNA virus that uses a reverse transcriptase to form DNA from RNA). The main target of HIV is the CD4 cell. The viral envelope protein, gp120, binds directly to the surface CD4 molecule and then expresses gp41. The virus enters the cell because of the interaction of cell surface and gp41. CCR5 is a chemokine receptor that functions as a coreceptor that enables HIV to gain access into macrophages. Like CD4, CCR5 is a receptor for several normal immune mediators. Initial infection may be through the macrophage by binding the CD4 and CCR5 surface molecules. The CD4+ T cell becomes infected by HIV-1 via cell surface CD4 and CXCR4 molecules. It has been speculated that there is another mechanism of entry into cells, as not all cells that become infected with HIV have had CD4 identified on their surface.

The effect of the virus is to destroy CD4 cells. This results in a progressive T-cell defect, with a spectrum of infections that is similar to that seen in congenital T-cell defects. Opportunistic infections and weaker pathogens are typical organisms to cause infection. There is poor regulation and clearing of malignant cells. Tumors that are usually slow-growing or benign, such as Kaposi's sarcoma, become rapidly malignant.

Clinical Features

General. The disease may lie dormant for many years.

Weight loss is a common feature of HIV infection, often because of gastrointestinal disease with diarrhea is often the cause of slower weight loss.

Infections. The key finding in AIDS is a pattern of infections that is similar to other T-cell deficient diseases. Unusual organisms such as *Pneumocystis carinii* or atypical mycobacteria are the cause of refractory pneumonia. Bacterial pneumonia is often due to *Pneumococci* and *Haemophilus influenzae*. *Mycobacterium tuberculosis* is often found in this population. A positive PPD may be present, but individuals are often anergic. MAC is a group of mycobacteria that can cause disseminated disease with fever, night sweats, diarrhea, weight loss, and abdominal pain in AIDS patients. Diarrhea is common for a number of reasons, such parasites (*Isospora belli*, *Giardia lamblia*, and *Entamoeba histolytica*), infestations (*Giardia lamblia*), or infections (rotavirus). Cryptosporidium organisms cause abdominal cramping, and watery, foul smelling stools. More common enteropathogens, *Salmonella*, *Shigella* and *E. coli* should also be considered.

Persistent candidal esophagitis is seen particularly in children and infants.

Neoplasms. There is an increase in the risk of malignancies, possibly because of activation of oncogenes and latent viruses. The malignancies that are noted include Kaposi's Sarcoma, non-Hodgkin's lymphoma, and cervical carcinoma, which may also define the condition. Cervical carcinomas is particularly frequent in adolescent girls.

Neurologic manifestations. Viral meningitis or encephalitis and peripheral neuropathies may occur at any stage of the disease. Opportunistic meningitis may occur with toxoplasma or cryptococcus. Central nervous lymphoma is also seen more frequently than in uninfected individuals. Progressive multifocal demyelinating leukoencephalopathy is a result of human polyomavirus infection. Autoimmune responses to virus in macrophages, CMV infection, therapy with nucleoside reverse transcriptase inhibitors or the HIV can cause peripheral neuropathy. Twenty percent of patients with advanced HIV infection develop AIDS dementia complex that includes poor concentration, problems with short-term memory, slowing of thought processes, motor incoordination, gait incoordination, and social withdrawal.

Wasting. Severe weight loss is a common feature of late HIV infection. Cachexia is related to secondary infection or to gastrointestinal disease, but anorexia is common during secondary infections. Reduced caloric intake is a major reason for the severe weight loss. Side effects from medication is a serious problem as well.

Immune parameters

Immunoglobulins. Early in the disease, patients have elevated immunoglobulins and hyperactive B cells. Typical levels may be as high as IgG = 2000 mg/dL (normal adult level 600 mg/dL). Much of this immunoglobulin is specific for HIV or is abnormal and does not have specific function.

Lymphocytes. Lymphopenia occurs progressively and is a reflection of disease severity.

Lymphocyte surface marker assessment by flow cytometry demonstrated loss of CD4 cells, with reversal of the normal CD4:CD8 ratio from 2:1 to 1:1 or 0.5:1. The absolute CD4+ count of less than $200/\mu L$ <14% of total lymphocytes is diagnostic of AIDS.

Transmission

The main route of transmission is intimate contact with blood and body fluids, most usually by sexual contact and the sharing of needles by IV drug abusers. Sexual transmission can occur through both heterosexual and homosexual contact. Initially, the predominant transmission was male homosexual intercourse, but presently, the predominant worldwide mode of transmission is heterosexual. Persons at risk for parenteral transmission include health care workers and people receiving unscreened blood transfusions.

The risk for health care workers is actually low and the average risk of infection for a needle stick is approximately 0.3%, dependent on the viral load in the contaminated material. The combination of Zidovudine, Lamivudine, and Indinavir is recommended for percutaneous exposure to infected blood as a prophylactic measure.

Prophylactic therapy to the infected mother with Zidovudine therapy has been shown to reduce the transmission rate from 25 to 8%.

Therapy

General therapy. As for any T-cell defect, active infections should be vigorously treated. Prophylaxis to prevent infections with PCP is essential to prevent severe pneumonia. The recommended approach is to use trimethoprim-sulfamethoxazole (150 mg trimethroprim/m^2/day with 750 mg sulfamethoxazole/m^2/day) administered orally in divided doses twice a day three times per week on consecutive days. Aerosolized pentamidine (300 mg via Respirgard II inhaler monthly) for those 5 years or older or daily oral dapsone (2 mg/kg, not to exceed 100 mg) are alternatives.

Specific drugs. The major groups of drugs that are in use in restricting proliferation of HIV are outlined. The specific use of these and related drugs is complex and is beyond the scope of this chapter.

Antiviral agents

Fusion Inhibitors: These drugs prevent the virus from entering the T cell by blocking receptor fusion.

- Enfuvirtide (Fuzeon, T-20)

Nonnucleoside Reverse Transcriptase Inhibitors (NNRTIs): This class of drugs functions by blocking nonnucleoside reverse transcriptase. Reverse transcriptase is an essential enzyme for HIV to make more copies of itself.

- Delavirdine (Rescriptor)
- Efavirenz (Sustiva)
- Nevirapine (Viramune)

Nucleoside/Nucleotide Reverse Transcriptase Inhibitors (NRTIs): Since HIV is a retrovirus, it requires reverse transcriptase to make a DNA copy of itself and replicate in the cell. These drugs reduce replication of the virus.

- Abacavir (Ziagen)
- Abacavir + Lamivudine + Zidovudine (Trizivir)
- Didanosine (Videx, ddI)
- Emtricitabine (Emtriva, FTC)
- Lamivudine (Epivir, 3TC)
- Lamivudine + Zidovudine (Combivir)
- Stavudine (Zerit, d4T)
- Tenofovir DF (Viread)
- Zalcitabine (HIVID, ddC)
- Zidovudine (Retrovir, AZT, ZDV)

Protease Inhibitors (PIs): This category of antiviral agents is specifically an inhibitor of the HIV protease. They bind to the active site of HIV-1 protease and prevent the processing of viral polyprotein precursors, resulting in the formation of immature noninfectious viral particles.

- Amprenavir (Agenerase)
- Atazanavir (Reyataz)
- Fosamprenavir (Lexiva, 908)
- Indinavir (Crixivan
- Lopinavir + Ritonavir (Kaletra)
- Nelfinavir (Viracept)
- Ritonavir (Norvir)
- Saquinavir (Fortovase, Invirase)

MISCELLANEOUS SECONDARY IMMUNE DEFECTS

Many chronic conditions have reduced immune function. These are noted in Table 10-8.

TABLE 10-8

CHRONIC DISEASES THAT HAVE INCIDENTAL IMMUNE DEFECTS

	CMI	CH50	Ig	Spleen	PMN	Mucosa
Diabetes	↓↓	–	–	–	–	↓
Sickle cell disease	–	–	–	↓↓↓	–	–
Immunosuppression	↓↓	–	↓	↓	↓↓	↓
Uremia	↓	–	–	↓	–	–
Nephrotic syndrome	–	↓	↓	–	–	–

Note: The immune alteration in common chronic diseases involve numerous aspects of immune function. These are CMI: cell mediated immunity (T-cell function); CH50 is a measure of complement function; Ig: immune globulin; PMN: polymorphonuclear cells; mucosa represents cutaneous and mucosal immune function.

Spleen

Patients who lose splenic function from splenectomy from surgery or autosplenectomy in sickle cell disease, are prone to infections with *Haemophilus* and *Pneumococcus*. Where the spleen is lost from trauma, there is no increase in infection risk, but for sickle cell disease or splenectomy for malignancy, the risk is very high.

KNOWN GENETIC DEFECTS

The genetic basis of several immune defects has been delineated. These are presented in Table 10-9. For many of these defects, the protein or enzyme that is affected by the abnormal gene is known.

TABLE 10-9

KNOWN GENETIC BASIS FOR IMMUNE DEFECTS IS PRESENTED, WITH THE PROTEIN OR ENZYME DEFECT WHERE IT IS KNOWN

Disease	Chromosome Locus	Protein Defect
Bruton's agammaglobulinemia	Xq22	B-cell specific tyrosine kinase
Hyper IgM	Xq26-27	qp39
Common variable	?6p21.3	Unknown
Selective IgA	?6p21.3	Unknown
Selective IgG	2p11;14q32.3	Unknown
XLP	Xq25-26	Unknown
Di George	22q11	Submicroscopic deletions
SCIDS	Xq13.1-21.1	Unknown
ADA	20qter	Adenosine deaminase
PNP	14q3.1	Nucleoside phosphorylase
Wiskott-Aldrich	Xp11-11.3	Unknown
Ataxia Telangiectasia	11q22.3	Unknown
LAD	21q22.3	Abnormal CD18

Suggested Reading

Bonilla, F. A. and R. S. Geha (2003). 12. Primary immunodeficiency diseases [erratum appears in J Allergy Clin Immunol 2003 Aug;112(2):267]. *J Allergy Clin Immunol* **111**(2 Suppl.): S571–81.

Buckley, R. H. (2002). Primary cellular immunodeficiencies. *J Allergy Clin Immunol* **109**(5): 747–57.

Elder, M. E. (2000). T-cell immunodeficiencies. *Pediatr Clin North Am* **47**(6): 1253–74.

Fischer, A. (2001). Primary T-lymphocyte immunodeficiencies. *Clin Rev Allergy Immunol* **20**(1): 3–26.

Fischer, A. (2002). Primary immunodeficiency diseases: natural mutant models for the study of the immune system. *Scand J Immunol* **55**(3): 238–41.

Frank, M. M. (2000). Complement deficiencies. *Pediatr Clin North Am* **47**(6): 1339–54.

Sorensen, R. U. and C. Moore (2000). Antibody deficiency syndromes. *Pediatr Clin North Am* **47**(6): 1225–52.

11

PRACTICAL PULMONARY FUNCTION STUDIES

FUNCTIONS OF THE LUNGS

The lungs are involved in vital functions that are available for assessment by specialized studies.

- Gas exchange
- Toxin removal
- Enzyme function
- Cardiovascular effects
- Cardiac filling
- Stroke volume
- Pulsus paradoxus
- Immune function

Pulmonary functions studies, as the only objective measurement, are the most valuable means of assessing severity, control, and chronicity of lung diseases. There are three key parameters that are measured by pulmonary function tests (PFT):

- Airflow
- Lung volumes
- Diffusing capacity

BASIC METHODOLOGY

A forced vital capacity (FVC) is the basis of all pulmonary functions. This test is performed by having the patient take a full inspiration, and then exhale as fast and as long as possible. The patient should exhale forcefully and hold expiration for a full 6 seconds. The held expiration ensures that the patient attains functional residual capacity (FRC) (see below). Exhalation is recorded as volume in liters and flow rate as liters per second. The key measurements are displayed in Figures 11-1 and 11-2. It is worth keeping in mind that PFTs are very effort dependent.

Detection of Flow

The most common device that is used is a pneumotachograph. This instrument is a flow sensor that functions by detecting changes in pressure across a membrane. The change in pressure is proportional to the flow rate. There are several variants on this method. Some are based on the fall in temperature across a heated wire or the movement of a turbine. Advances in electronic have improved the accuracy of these methods. With refined electronic corrections, the inevitable drift in the system can be removed from calculations.

Measurement of Flow

Flow is measured and expressed on two types of curve. The first plots time in seconds against volume in liters (time-volume), and is a measure of the

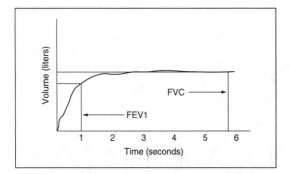

FIGURE 11-1

A PLOT OF TIME AGAINST VOLUME REPRESENT-ING FORCED EXHALATION.

The patient exhales from maximal inhalation to maximal exhalation as forcefully as possible. Exhalation should be held for six to eight seconds. The significance of these measurements is presented in Table 11-1 and in the text.

portion of the vital capacity that is exhaled at time points. The second plots volume in liters against flow rate in liters per second, and is a reflection of the rate of flow at different lung volumes.

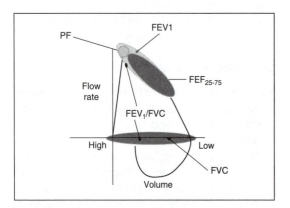

FIGURE 11-2

SPIROMETRIC TRACING SHOWING THE COMPO-NENTS OF THE NORMAL FLOW-VOLUME LOOP.

The significance of these components is explained in Table 11-1 and in the text. The origin of the X axis represents maximal inhalation, and therefore high lung volumes and the end of the X axis scale is low lung volume, representative of FRC. This loop is the basis of evaluating flow parameters of lung function. PF = peak flow, representing large airways; FEF 25–75 = forced expiratory flow from 25% to 75% of FVC, representing small to medium airways.

Time-Volume Curve

An example of this type of curve is shown in Figure 11-1.

There are two key measurements derived from this graph.

FVC is the total volume of air that is exhaled from maximal inhalation to maximal exhalation. This measurement is the basis for most of the lung assessments described.

Forced expiratory volume in 1 second (FEV1) is a sensitive measure of airflow out of the lung. It is the volume of air that is exhaled in the first second, as illustrated in Figure 11-1. The FEV1 is normally >85% of FVC.

The ratio of FEV1/FVC is used as the standard measure of airway obstruction. It is expressed as a percentage (Figure 11-1).

Flow-Volume Curve

An example of this type of curve is shown in Figure 11-2.

In this type of graph, the FVC appears on the X axis. The shape of the curve represents the rate of flow at different lung volumes. From the origin, the Y axis shows the fastest rate of flow, which represents the peak flow (PF). This region is marked in Figure 11-2. The rate of flow then falls as the volume of the lungs decreases. The small airways then empty simultaneously causing a brief rise in flow rate, producing a typical appearance of the curve. The FEV1 is shown on this curve in Figure 11-2. The forced expiratory flow (FEF) 25–75% is a measurement that is reflective of flow from the small airways and integrates the flow rates from 75 to 25% of the FVC. The FEF 25–75% is the only portion of the curve that is effort independent. The FEV1/FVC ratio is indicated on the curve in Figure 11-2 (Table 11-1).

Volume

The basis of assessment of lung volumes is the total lung capacity (TLC). The total lung capacity and volume subdivisions are illustrated in Figure 11-3.

TABLE 11-1

THE COMPONENTS OF THE FLOW-VOLUME LOOP THAT CONSTITUTE SPIROMETRY

Forced expiratory volume in 1 second (FEV1)	Volume that is exhaled in the first second in liters per second. This region of the curve represents large to medium sized airways
FEV1/FVC ratio	This is an important measure of airflow out of the lungs. It is normally greater than 85%
Peak expiratory flow rate (PEFR) (or peak flow—PF)	Measures the most rapid flow of air, and reflects the larger airways
Forced expiratory flow from 25 to 75 % of FVC (FEF 25–75%)	Measures flow rate in the midportion of the FVC; reflective of flow in the mid- to small-sized airways.

Note: These values are reflective of airflow. They are shown pictorially in the graph in Figure 11-2 as well. They are derived by the patient exhaling forcefully into the flow sensor. The volume and flow are taken from maximal inhalation to maximal exhalation.

Volume Measurements Are Made Using Three Methods

Body Plethysmography

A plethysmograph is a chamber that seals tightly and can detect small changes in volume. The patient breathes into a mouthpiece and various maneuvers, such as panting and forced exhalation are employed. The measurements are derived from the flow curve and direct volume measurements. This technique is effort dependent, and requires comprehension on the part of the patient to understand the demands of the test.

Nitrogen Washout Test

The patient breathes through a one-way valve that is attached to but not yet connected to a reservoir filled with 100% O_2 or a demand valve connected to a pressurized O_2 source. At the end of a normal resting expiration the valve is opened, allowing the patient to breathe through the one-way valve. Expired nitrogen is measured at the mouth. Inspired or expired minute ventilations are measured continuously. Test continues until exhaled N_2 concentrations fall <2%, indicating a "washout" of communicating airways and alveoli. Total inhaled volume and final N_2 concentration can be used to calculate the FRC. Computerized systems calculate FRC with each breath and adjust calculated value after each subsequent breath. This test has the added advantage that it measures alveolar volume as well.

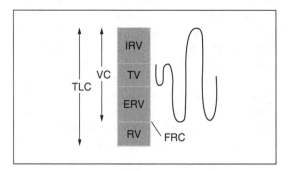

FIGURE 11-3

REPRESENTATION OF THE LUNG VOLUME SUB-DIVISIONS.

The significance is discussed in Table 11-2 and in the text. TLC: total lung capacity; VC: vital capacity; RV: residual volume; ERV: expiratory reserve volume; IRV: inspiratory reserve volume; TV: tidal volume; FRC: functional residual capacity.

Helium Dilution Test

For this test, the patient breathes through a valve that is open to room air but connected to a reservoir (spirometer) containing 5–10% helium.

TABLE 11-2

PRESENTATION OF COMPONENTS OF LUNG VOLUME MEASUREMENTS

Forced vital capacity (FVC)	Volume in liters from maximal inhalation to maximal forced exhalation
Slow vital capacity (SVC)	Volume in liters from maximal inhalation to maximal slow exhalation. In the presence of obstruction, SVC is higher than FVC because the airways close earlier with FVC
Total lung capacity (TLC)	Measures total lung volume
Residual volume (RV)	The volume of air that is left in the lungs after maximal exhalation, usually 20%
RV/TLC ratio	Increased in asthma because of air trapping

Note: These values are reflective of airflow. They are shown pictorially in the graph in Figure 11-3 as well.

At the end of a normal resting expiration (FRC) the valve is opened allowing the patient to breathe from the reservoir. Carbon dioxide is chemically scrubbed from the rebreathing circuit and oxygen is added to keep the end expiratory level constant. The test continues until the concentration of helium in the system is constant (<0.02% change in helium concentration) for a minimum of 15 seconds. Initial and final helium concentrations, the volume of helium and air added to the system, and the system dead space can then be used to calculate the volume added to the system to achieve that dilution (FRC).

Significance of the Volume Measurements

Total lung capacity (TLC) represents the full intrathoracic volume. It is reduced in restrictive disease.

Slow vital capacity (SVC) is the same measurement as the FVC, but it is measured at a comfortable exhalation pace. Discrepancy between the FVC and SVC is indicative of unequal gas distribution in the lung and airway obstruction.

The residual volume (RV) is a measurement of the volume that remains in the lungs at the end of expiration. It is essential for normal respiration. It is increased in obstructive lung diseases.

The ratio RV/TLC is useful to express the degree of air trapping present. Normally, RV is 20% of TLC.

The components of lung volume measurements and their significance are presented in Table 11-2.

BRONCHIAL CHALLENGE

In cases where the diagnosis of asthma may be in doubt, a challenge test is used. Methacholine is regarded as the "gold standard" to diagnose asthma where the diagnosis may be in doubt. Methacholine is an acetylcholine analog that will cause bronchoconstriction. Asthmatics are more sensitive than controls by 10-fold or greater. Methacholine is inhaled in increasing total dose using a precise dosimeter, and spirometry is monitored. A fall in FEV1 of 20% or greater is diagnostic. The result is presented as the PC20, which is the cumulative dose needed to cause a 20% fall in FEV1.

Other bronchoconstrictive agents may be used, including histamine, adenosine, specific antigen, cold air, and distilled water. Exercise is a commonly used challenge, delivered in a controlled manner via a treadmill or a bicycle ergometer.

DIFFUSION STUDIES

Diffusion measurements are essentially an assessment of the rate of transfer of O_2 across the alveolar capillary gap. Carbon monoxide is used as a surrogate for O_2, as it has similar transfer and binding characteristics.

There are two key differences which should be kept in mind when interpreting results of CO diffusion. First, CO is approximately 25-fold more soluble than O_2, and its diffusion is not rate limited. Second, CO has a higher binding coefficient to hemoglobulin than O_2. The actual technique that is used is similar to helium dilution. The patient inhales from a bag containing a known concentration of CO. The difference between starting and ending concentrations is calculated as liters/min and corrected for lung volume.

Clinical Evaluation of Diffusion

A good clinical assessment of diffusion of O_2 can be obtained by two methods. Both require that arterial blood gasses be drawn from the patient.

Breathing 100% O_2

If a patient is given 100% O_2 to breathe at sea level, the PaO_2 (blood oxygen) should be 630 torr. If the patient has a lower PaO_2, there is a diffusion gradient present. This method is useful for small children and infants who are unable to perform pulmonary function studies. Finding a gradient indicates that there is disease present that involves the alveolar capillary space. This gap is normally only a few

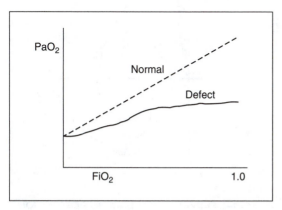

FIGURE   11-4

A CLINICAL ASSESSMENT OF A PATIENT WITH A DIFFUSION DEFECT.

At an FiO_2 1.0 (100% O_2) the PaO_2 is half normal, indicating a severe diffusion defect.

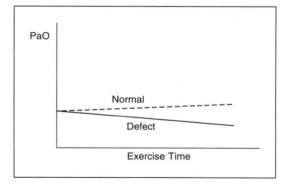

FIGURE   11-5

A CLINICAL ASSESSMENT OF A PATIENT WITH A DIFFUSION DEFECT.

When the patient exercises, there is a fall in PaO_2 compared to the control, indicating a diffusion defect.

Angstroms wide. If it is increased, the O_2 takes too long to cross, and does not attach to a red cell. This type of interstitial lung disease can be caused by infection, inflammatory diseases such as rheumatoid diseases and malignancies.

Figure 11-4 illustrates the clinical application of this test.

Exercise

The patient is asked to exercise, and PaO_2 is measured. Normally, the PaO_2 should be maintained, even with vigorous exercise. If there is a diffusion defect present, the PaO_2 will fall (Figure 11-5).

CLINICAL SIGNIFICANCE OF PFT

There are essentially three types of defects that may be seen in the lungs. All three are detectable by pulmonary function studies. These are obstructive, restrictive, and diffusional.

Obstructive

These are conditions that block passage of air on exhalation.

Figure 11-6 presents a typical flow-volume loop in obstruction, and Table 11-3 depicts typical values in this group of conditions.

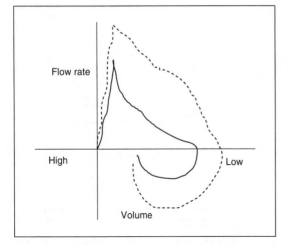

FIGURE 11-6

A TYPICAL FLOW-VOLUME LOOP IN OBSTRUCTION.

A typical obstructive pattern is shown in the solid line. The dashed line is the normal for comparison. The flow loop shows a typical "scooped" appearance, and a lower FVC is reflected on the *X* axis. Table 11-3 shows the matching values for this loop.

TABLE 11-3

VALUES OF PFT PARAMETERS COMMONLY SEEN IN *OBSTRUCTIVE DISEASE*

	% Predicted	Interpretation
FVC	75	Reduced
SVC	85	Less reduced
PEEF	70	Reduced
FEV1	60–70	Reduced
FEV1/FVC	70	Reduced
FEF 25–75%	55	Reduced
TLC	100	Normal
RV	35	Increased

Note: This table complements Figure 11-6. There is a reduction of FVC, while SVC is less reduced and nearly normal. This pattern indicates that there is unequal gas distribution throughout the lungs. Residual volume is increased, reflecting air trapping from the obstructive disease. PEEF is reduced, as is FEV1, reflective of the degree of obstruction. There is more severe reduction in flow in the small airways, in FEF 25–75%. FEV1/FVC ratio is reduced.

Examples of obstructive disease include the following:

- Asthma
- Bronchopulmonary dysplasia
- Chronic obstructive pulmonary disease
- Rheumatoid diseases
- Cystic fibrosis

Restrictive Conditions

These conditions cause a reduction in the total lung capacity.

Figure 11-7 presents a typical flow-volume loop in restriction and Table 11-4 depicts typical values in this group of conditions.

Examples of this condition include the following:

- Pulmonary fibrosis
- Collagen-vascular disease
- Cystic fibrosis
- Hypersensitivity lung disease

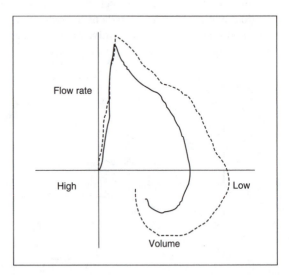

FIGURE 11-7

A TYPICAL FLOW-VOLUME LOOP IN RESTRICTION.

Typical restrictive pattern is shown in the solid line. The dashed line is the normal for comparison. Note the low FVC, represented by the narrowed flow volume loop. The contour of the loop is similar to the normal pattern, indicating normal airflow.

TABLE 11-4

VALUES ON PFT COMMONLY SEEN IN RESTRICTIVE DISEASE

	% Predicted	Interpretation
FVC	70	Reduced
SVC	70	Reduced
PEEF	100	Normal
FEV1	>95	Normal
FEV1/FVC	>90	Normal
FEF 25–75%	80–100	Normal
TLC	70	Reduced
RV	100	Normal

Note: FVC and SVC are equally reduced. TLC is also decreased, but residual volume is normal in proportion to the reduction of TLC. Flow parameters, FEV1, FEV1/FVC, and FEF 25–75% are normal.

TABLE 11-5

VALUES ON PFT COMMONLY SEEN IN *MIXED OBSTRUCTIVE AND RESTRICTIVE DISEASE*

	% Predicted	Interpretation
FVC	70	Reduced
SVC	75	Reduced
PEEF	65	Reduced
FEV1	65	Reduced
FEV1/FVC	70	Reduced
FEF 25–75%	45	Reduced
TLC	75	Reduced
RV	40	Increased

Note: Flow parameters are all reduced (PEEF, FEV1, FEV1/FVC, and FEF 25–75%), unlike pure restrictive disease (Table 11-4). Lung volumes are all reduced, except for RV, indicating air trapping. This is typical of chronic obstructive lung diseases.

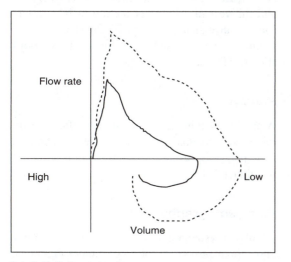

FIGURE 11-8

TYPICAL MIXED OBSTRUCTIVE AND RESTRICTIVE PATTERN.

Typical mixed obstructive and restrictive pattern is shown in the solid line. The dashed line is the normal for comparison. Note the "scooped" appearance to the flow-volume loop, indicative of obstruction. In addition, the FVC, as represented on the X axis is reduced. Volume measurements are needed to determine whether a concomitant restrictive disease is present. These values are shown in Table 11-5.

- Pulmonary hemorrhage
- Muscle weakness

Mixed Pattern

A combination of diseases, such as asthma and rheumatoid arthritis, can produce a mixed picture on pulmonary function. An example is seen in Figure 11-8 (Table 11-5).

Diffusional

In these conditions, there is reduced transfer of oxygen across the alveolar capillary gap and resultant hypoxemia.

Examples of this type of defect are the following:

- Interstitial lung disease
- Hyaline membrane disease
- High altitude
- Pulmonary fibrosis

INFANT PFT

It is not possible to perform standard PFTs on infants and young children. There are four methods that have evolved to investigate infant PFT.

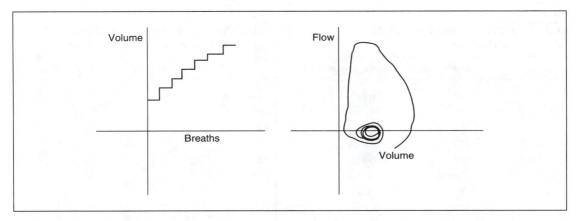

FIGURE 11-9

DEFLATION LOOP IN AN INFANT.

The stacking of breath is seen on the left, and the resultant loop on the right.

Deflation Loop

This method involves having the infant wear a tight mask. When the infant exhales, a shutter is closed, stacking breaths forcing an increase in residual volume. At maximal inhalation, the shutter is released, creating a pseudo forced loop (Figure 11-9).

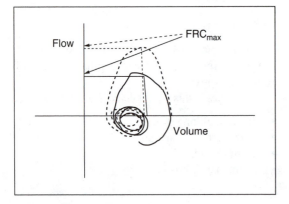

FIGURE 11-10

SQUEEZE LOOP.

Normal control is shown as a dotted line and an infant with BPD and airflow obstruction in a solid line. The two curves are compared at FRC_{max}.

Squeeze Loop

A tight fitting vest is placed on a sedated infant, and the vest in inflated at the top of inspiration, forcing an exhalation loop. FRCmax is a measurement that is used to compare flow loops (Figure 11-10).

Passive

A passive loop is measured with the infant breathing at tidal breaths. This is not a useful technique, as it may miss even severe obstruction. It is not recommended.

Plethysmography

Infant plethysmographs have been developed. They allow the measurement of lung volumes in infants.

DYNAMIC MEASUREMENTS

- Lung resistance
  Measures the impairment to flow of air
- Lung compliance
  Measures the elasticity of the lungs
- Lung conductance
  Measures the ease of airflow

Suggested Reading

Anees, W. (2003). Use of pulmonary function tests in the diagnosis of occupational asthma. *Ann Allergy Asthma Immunol* **90**(5 Suppl. 2): 47–51.

Crapo, R. O. and R. L. Jensen (2003). Standards and interpretive issues in lung function testing. *Respir Care* **48**(8): 764–72.

Evans, S. E. and P. D. Scanlon (2003). Current practice in pulmonary function testing. *Mayo Clin Proc* **78**(6): 758–63; quiz 763.

Fauroux, B. (2003). Respiratory muscle testing in children. *Paediatr Respir Rev* **4**(3): 243–9.

Ferguson, G. T., P. L. Enright, et al. (2000). Office spirometry for lung health assessment in adults: a consensus statement from the National Lung Health Education Program. *Respir Care* **45**(5): 513–30.

Frey, U., J. Stocks, et al. (2000). Specifications for equipment used for infant pulmonary function testing.

ERS/ATS Task Force on Standards for Infant Respiratory Function Testing. European Respiratory Society/American Thoracic Society [comment]. *Eur Respir J* **16**(4): 731–40.

Gruffydd-Jones, K. (2002). Measuring pulmonary function in practice. *Practitioner* **246**(1635): 445–9.

Klug, B. H. (2002). Evaluation of some techniques for measurements of lung function in young children. *Dan Med Bull* **49**(3): 227–41.

Sharp, J. K. (2002). Monitoring early inflammation in CF. Infant pulmonary function testing. *Clin Rev Allergy Immunol* **23**(1): 59–76.

Weiner, D. J., J. L. Allen, et al. (2003). Infant pulmonary function testing. *Curr Opin Pediatr* **15**(3): 316–22.

Winkelman, J. W. and M. J. Tanasijevic (2002). Noninvasive testing in the clinical laboratory. *Clin Lab Med* **22**(2): 547–58.

12

INVESTIGATION OF ALLERGIES

The history of symptoms and a pattern of allergic reactions are essential in evaluating a possible allergic condition. Investigative tools have limited validity unless they are correlated with the history. A positive test that has no bearing on the patient's clinical responses should be disregarded, irrespective of the method used. The techniques available depend on detecting the consequences of an allergic reaction.

MEASURABLE CONSEQUENCES OF AN ALLERGIC REACTION

Eosinophilia

Eosinophils will increase in response to an allergic stimulus, because there is release of eosinophil chemoattractants during an allergic response. This increase is local, in tissues, and in peripheral blood. There is a large list of causes of eosinophilia (Table 12-1), so the finding of elevated eosinophils is not particularly helpful in isolation. The presence of eosinophilia should be taken in the context of the patient's history. The significance of elevation of blood eosinophils is unclear.

There may be a local increase in eosinophils, e.g., nasal secretions, bronchial washings, or in biopsy specimens. Nasal eosinophilia is helpful in differentiating allergic rhinitis from other causes. The only other condition that causes an increase in nasal eosinophils is eosinophilic rhinitis. The technique involves taking a blown specimen, making a smear of the mucus, and staining with a white cell stain (Wright-Giemsa). More than 20% eosinophils (some authors have used 10%) are regarded as a positive test in adults. In children greater than 4% is taken as positive.

Tissue eosinophils accumulate for a number of reasons, and their presence does not diagnose allergies. Pulmonary eosinophils are found in eosinophilic pneumonia, idiopathic eosinophilia, and hypereosinophilic syndromes, malignancies especially Hodgkin's lymphoma and parasitic infections. In children, visceral lava migrans, caused by toxocara infestation, causes eosinophilic pulmonary infiltrates that are transient and shifting. Eosinophilic infiltrates can occur into stomach and esophagus. The cause can relate to food allergies, but is more often idiopathic (Table 12-2).

TABLE 12-1

CAUSES OF EOSINOPHILIA

Atopic
  Rhinitis
    Allergic
    Eosinophilic
  Asthma
  Food and drug allergies

Malignancy
  Hypereosinophilic syndromes (premalignant)
  Leukemia
  Lymphomas (especially Hodgkin's)
  Mastocytosis

Infections
  Parasitic infections
    Ascaris
    Toxocara
  Fungal infections

Rheumatologic
  Lupus erythematosus
  Rheumatoid arthritis
  Churg-Strauss vasculitis
  Polyarteritis nodosa

Immunologic
  Specific immune deficiency diseases
    Wiskott-Aldrich
  Transplant rejection

Note: This is a partial list containing more common causes.

TABLE 12-2

COMMONLY USED ANTIGENS IN ALLERGY SKIN TESTING

Indoor
  Animal dander
    Cat
    Dog
    Rodent
    Mouse
    Rat
    Hamster
  House dust mites
    Dermatophagoides farinae
    Dermatophagoides pteronyssinus
  Cockroach
  Molds and mold spores

Outdoor
  Pollens
    Region specific
  Trees
  Grass
  Weeds
    Ragweed
  Molds and mold spores

Food
  Dairy products
    Eggs
    Cow's milk
  Seafood
    Shrimp
    Crab
    Clams
    Oysters
  Fish
  Peanuts
    Tree nuts
    Pecans
    Cashew nuts
    Almonds
  Meats
  Potatoes

Measurement of IgE

IgE can be detected by in vivo and in vitro techniques. In vivo assessments are more reliable.

In Vivo

Allergy skin test. This test detects the presence of IgE that is bound to mast cells. It has the advantage of testing whether specific IgE is present, whether it will cause mast cells to degranulate and whether it will produce a wheal and flare response. Since the test is performed on the skin, an assumption is being made that the mast cells in the skin respond in the same way as mast cells in the lung, nasal mucosa, and gut. This is the least costly of the methods for detecting IgE. It should be interpreted by a trained physician and correlated with the patient's history. The patient has to be off of all antihistamines for allergy skin test. First generation sedating antihistamines (diphenhydramine, hydroxyzine) should be stopped for 72 hours prior to testing. The long-acting, nonsedating drugs (desloratadine, cetirizine, fexofenadine) should be stopped for a week before testing is done.

Methods. There are three methods of introducing the antigen into the skin.

> Scratch: superficial to 1 mm into the epidermis.
> Skin prick: 1–2 mm into the epidermis.
> Intradermal: injection of 20 μL into the epidermis; 500–1000-fold more sensitive than scratch or prick methods.

Technique. The antigen is dissolved in a 50% glycerol solution for scratch and prick tests. Traditionally, a 20-μL drop is placed on the forearm and the skin is scarified under the drop. A scarification needle is used to make the scratches.

Using a prick method is easier and does not require as much skill and training to get uniform results. There are two approaches: placing the drop on the skin and puncturing through it, as with the scratch test, or using a device to carry the drop and puncture the skin in one movement.

- Bifurcated needle: this is the standard method for the prick test, but it difficult to use consistently and obtain uniform results. The technician must be carefully trained in its use.
- Multitest: an eight armed unit with 2 mm prongs on each arm. Each antigen is loaded onto one of the prongs. The unit is then pressed evenly onto the forearm or back (in small children). If two units are used, one can test 14 common antigens and a positive and negative control. This is the ideal method, especially for children. It is nearly painless and rapid. It can be applied uniformly with minimal training. The apparatus will also accommodate filling wells in a loading tray with the antigens and controls. The multitest is then fully loaded by

placing it in the wells. This will allow rapid testing in a busy allergy office.

Intradermal. Twenty microliters of an aqueous solution of the antigen is injected into the epidermis on the forearm, raising a small area. For intradermal testing, the solution does not contain glycerin.

Controls

> Positive: histamine
> Negative: antigen solvent

Antigens

There are three main groups of antigens that are commonly used, though there is overlap among them. They can be considered as indoor, outdoor, and food allergens. They are shown in Table 12-2.

Interpretation

The test is evaluated by the presence of a weal and flare response at the site of antigen placement.

A positive test is read as 3 mm larger than the negative control; a size equal to the positive control is regarded as 3+ positive. For a more accurate assessment, the wheal is traced and the area is calculated. The size of the wheal can also be recorded as the two maximal diameters.

This test is only semiquantitative, and the size of the wheal does not correlate closely with the severity of the allergic reaction, other than that a large reaction is more likely to be associated with a more severe clinical reaction.

Intradermal tests are oversensitive, increasing the risk of a false positive. They are generally used to detect other sensitivities in patients who will receive immunotherapy (see Chap. 16).

Interpretation must be carefully correlated with history. Testing for environmental antigens is sensitive, and there is a good correlation with history. Some available antigens are shown in Table 12-2. There is a strong seasonal pattern in the northern part of the United States. The pattern blurs in the south, as the seasons tend to overlap more. Trees tend to pollinate in the spring, grass grows and pollinates throughout the summer and weeds, especially ragweed, pollinates in the fall. Outdoor molds are more

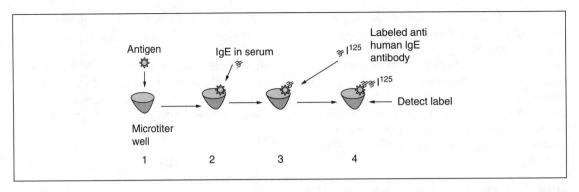

F I G U R E   1 2 - 1

METHOD OF RAST.

(1) Antigen is added to solid medium, in this case a microtiter well. (2) The patient's serum is added and specific IgE binds to the adsorbed antigen. (3) Labeled anti-IgE is added. The label may be a radiolabel, ELISA, or chemiluminescence. This antibody binds to the patient's IgE that is bound to adsorbed antigen. (4) The concentration of label is assessed by the appropriate method. The amount of specific IgE present in patient's serum is in keeping with the count of the amount of label present.

prevalent in the fall as well, and decaying leaves provide a large reservoir of mold spores and hyphae.

Testing for foods is more difficult to interpret. There is a high frequency of false positive tests, and a positive test without a supporting history of reactions to the food is not meaningful. There is a 55–65% predictive value of food testing for a positive result, which is not much better than a random chance distribution. On the other hand, there is a 95% predictive value for a negative result. Allergy testing for foods is most helpful for excluding a food as a cause of a reaction such as urticaria. A negative test will exclude a suspected food, such as milk, as a cause of the allergic response. The patient can cautiously eat the food where there is a negative food allergy test.

In Vitro

Total IgE. The measurement of total IgE in serum is of limited value. Having an increase in total IgE implies that there is atopy present, but clinical confirmation is needed for an elevated titer.

Specific IgE. There are several versions of in vitro tests, but they are all based on the same principle; only the detection method changes (Figure 12-1).

The antigen is bound to an absorptive surface such as paper or plastic. The antigen is adsorbed onto the surface, and nonspecific binding is prevented with albumin or other protein that will not react with IgE. The plate is then incubated with the patient's serum, when specific IgE binds to the antigen. Rabbit or mouse IgG that has antihuman IgE specificity is then added and incubated. The amount of anti-IgE that binds to the plate reflects the concentration of specific IgE in the patients' serum. The IgE–anti-IgE complex on the paper disc is measured by a detection system that is added to the anti-IgE antibody. Detection systems that have been used include radiolabel with I^{125}, chemiluminescence or enzyme-linked immunosorbent assay (ELISA) systems. There is then a direct correlation between the level of IgE in patient's serum and the degree of positivity of the assay (disintegrations/min for radiolabel; color intensity for ELISA). The original method is the Radioallergosorbent test (RAST), which uses radiolabeling with I^{125}. Other detection systems are in use, and ELISA and chemiluminescence are frequent examples.

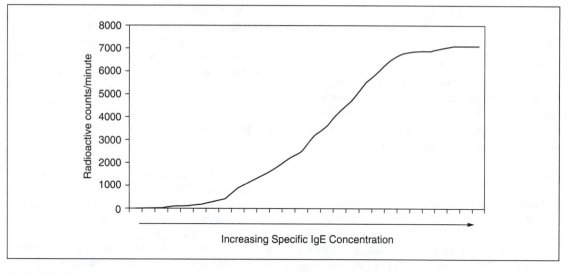

TYPICAL TITRATION CURVE FOR A RAST USING ¹²⁵I TO DETECT SPECIFIC IGE, DEPICTED ON THE X AXIS.

Radioactive counts are presented on the Y axis, but the appropriate units can be substituted depending on the detection system.

A representative titration curve is shown in Figure 12-2. Some newer systems such as CAP-RAST are better for children as they use less serum and are more sensitive.

This assay is actually limited in its clinical significance, although it sensitively measures specific IgE in at low serum concentrations.

Drawbacks of in vitro testing. The test only evaluates circulating antibody, and does not assess whether there is clinically relevant binding to mast cells. IgE only is clinically active when fixed to mast cells or basophils. RAST (or equivalent) only indicates that IgE is present in circulation. It does not indicate whether it will bind to mast cells, or whether it can trigger mast cell or basophil disintegration. Two extreme situations could arise theoretically. A false negative could result from the majority of specific IgE being bound to mast cells, reducing the level of circulating antibody below the threshold of detection. Equally, a strongly positive RAST may have little clinical significance because

IgE is all in circulation and has not bound to mast cells.

Indications for in vitro testing. The major indication for using in vitro tests is in the situation where the patient has a history of a strong reaction to an antigen, for example, anaphylaxis to peanut antigen and it would be dangerous to apply the antigen to the skin. The other situation where the blood test is preferable to prick skin test is where there is abnormal skin, because of atopic dermatitis. In young children (under 18 months) the prick skin test may not be reliable. Another situation where the skin test should be used is if the patient is unable to discontinue antihistamines because of ongoing symptoms.

An in vitro test is indicated where skin testing is unreliable or dangerous:

- Under 18 months of age.
- Extensive skin disorder, e.g., eczema.
- For antigens that may cause a systemic reaction, e.g., food or insect venoms where a history of a strong reaction is given.

CHALLENGE TESTS

Nasal

Patients may be challenged with antigen intranasally. The response is assessed clinically, by subjective impression of rhinorrhea and nasal congestion. Objective measurement is made by rhinomanometry, which quantifies nasal airflow. A positive reaction would demonstrate a reduction in airflow.

Inhaled

Inhalation antigen challenge is occasionally used in patients who have asthma to conform a reaction to an antigen. However, this tool is used more for research. The measurement is the dose that causes a 20% fall in FEV1, known as the PD20. Patients who are allergic to the antigen will reach PD20 sooner than those who are not allergic. There is a good correlation between the degree of sensitivity to the antigen, and how rapidly the patient will attain PD20.

Oral

The gold standard for food allergy is the blinded food challenge. The patient has a bland, nonallergenic diet for several days prior to testing. The offending food is given in an opaque capsule and the patient is observed for the development of gastrointestinal symptoms, urticaria or worsening of eczema. This technique is usually used as a research tool and is performed in a double-blinded design using an identical looking placebo control capsule.

SIGNIFICANCE OF ALLERGY TESTING

A positive history is 60% predictive of a positive allergy test result.

A negative history is 70% predictive of a negative result.

The history is most important in deciding whether to perform allergy skin testing on a patient or not. Another interpretation is that it is of little value to perform allergy testing on patients who do not give a history that is suggestive of atopy.

Suggested Reading

Baatjes, A. J., R. Sehmi, et al. (2002). Anti-allergic therapies: effects on eosinophil progenitors. *Pharmacol Ther* **95**(1): 63–72.

Brito-Babapulle, F. (2003). The eosinophilias, including the idiopathic hypereosinophilic syndrome. *Br J Haematol* **121**(2): 203–23.

Chapman, M. D., A. M. Smith, et al. (2000). Recombinant allergens for diagnosis and therapy of allergic disease. *J Allergy Clin Immunol* **106**(3): 409–18.

Dombrowicz, D. and M. Capron (2001). Eosinophils, allergy and parasites. *Curr Opin Immunol* **13**(6): 716–20.

Emanuel, I. A. (1998). In vitro testing for allergy diagnosis. Comparison of methods in common use. *Otolaryngol Clin North Am* **31**(1): 27–34.

Kay, A. B. and A. Menzies-Gow (2003). Eosinophils and interleukin-5: the debate continues [comment]. *Am J Respir Crit Care Med* **167**(12): 1586–7.

Moqbel, R. and P. Lacy (2000). Molecular mechanisms in eosinophil activation. *Chem Immunol* **78**: 189–98.

Prussin, C. and D. D. Metcalfe (2003). 4. IgE, mast cells, basophils, and eosinophils [erratum appears in J Allergy Clin Immunol 2003 Aug;112(2):267]. *J Allergy Clin Immunol* **111**(2 Suppl.): S486–94.

Scadding, G. K. (2001). Non-allergic rhinitis: diagnosis and management. *Curr Opin Allergy Clin Immunol* **1**(1): 15–20.

Valenta, R., P. Steinberger, et al. (1996). Immunological and structural similarities among allergens: prerequisite for a specific and component-based therapy of allergy. *Immunol Cell Biol* **74**(2): 187–94.

Valenta, R., S. Vrtala, et al. (1998). Recombinant allergens. *Allergy* **53**(6): 552–61.

13

MANAGEMENT OF IMMUNE DEFICIENCY AND RECURRENT INFECTIONS

Part I. Investigation

GENERAL

The range of causes of recurrent infections is broad. The investigation should be based on the history and the pattern of infections. Infections that occur at one particular site, such as the maxillary sinus cavities, strongly suggest a mechanical problem. In this case, procedures that delineate the site will be helpful in isolating the pathology.

X Ray

In general, x-ray studies are most helpful when used to answer a specific question. In recurrent infections, x rays can help with distinguishing acute problems, as pneumonia, and suggest a chronic source, as bronchiectasis. A chest radiograph in a patient who has otitis media and no pulmonary symptom is unlikely to be helpful.

Plain

Chest x ray

Acute. The striking acute features on chest radiograph may be pneumonia, a diffuse infiltrate, or patchy lesions. There may be narrowing apparent in a main bronchus, suggestive of obstruction. Unilateral hyperinflation may suggest a foreign body in an airway, usually a mainstem bronchus. There may be pneumonia distal to the site of obstruction. A barium swallow study is indicated if there is evidence to suggest a vascular ring or sling around the trachea or mainstem bronchus.

Chronic. Persistent diffuse infiltrates may be seen in pneumocystis infection, or CMV or other pulmonary inflammatory virus. The radiographic pattern alone is seldom diagnostic of a particular organism. An infiltrate that is persistent in a particular lobe, especially in the left lower lobe, is suggestive of a sequestered segment of the lung. This is a condition in which a lobe, or segment of a lobe fails to develop properly. There is a tenuous connection with the bronchi, and the segment derives its blood supply from the bronchial arteries, rather than the pulmonary. Gas exchange does not take place in this porion of the lung, and there is stasis because of the poor bronchial connection. The result is repeated infections in the same site. Confirmation is with a CT scan using vascular contrast.

Chronic aspiration gives rise to a typical pattern of persistent infiltrates in the upper lobes of the lungs. This is because aspiration occurs most while patients are supine, and the most direct path is to the upper lobes.

Another typical pattern that is seen on chest x ray is the appearance of streaky infiltrates in the upper lobes in a patient with persistent infections and an asthma like presentation. This appearance is seen with upper lobe collapse and bronchiectasis that is a diagnostic criterion for cystic fibrosis.

The possibility of a foreign body in the bronchi can be determined by fluoroscopy of the chest. This shows that there is uneven movement of the diaphragms, one diaphragm does not move or that there is paradoxical movement of one leaf of the diaphragm. A CT scan of the chest is confirmatory, if needed. A history of choking on food has the closest predictive value for aspiration of a foreign body. In adults, there is an increased risk of foreign body where alcoholism or drug use is present. In children, there is an association with mental retardation.

Sinuses. Plain x-ray views of the sinuses are of limited value. A PA view and Water's view (with the chin elevated to have a clear view of the maxillary sinuses) will help with the diagnosis of acute sinusitis. There is the appearance of cloudiness of the sinuses or complete opacification. An air-fluid level will indicate the possible presence of pus in the sinus cavity.

A CT scan in the coronal plane is the best approach if chronic sinus disease is suspected. This study will not only demonstrate the presence of fluid or pus, but can also reveal underlying anatomic abnormalities.

Sweat Chloride

Measurement of chloride levels in sweat is an established method of diagnosing cystic fibrosis and reflects the abnormal water transportation that is characteristic of the disease. The classical test is by sweat iontophoresis, but newer methods are becoming available. A minimum of 100 mg of sweat is needed for an accurate test. It is advisable to perform the test at a Cystic Fibrosis center where it is done frequently as there are many pitfalls in performing this test.

Patients who have recurrent infections involving the lungs, sinuses, and middle ear accompanied by weight loss, steatorrhea, and abdominal distension should have a sweat chloride measurement. Infants may present with meconium ileus and intestinal obstruction. The clinical features may be more subtle, and patients with cystic fibrosis may present with persistent pneumonia, without any other features of the disease.

pH Probe

Gastroesophageal reflux may be a silent cause of aspiration pneumonia. The gold standard for detecting reflux is the pH probe. This is a fine catheter with one pH meter at the end and a second higher up the catheter. When properly placed, the end pH probe is above the cardiac sphincter of the stomach, and the proximal one is just below the level of the vocal cords. In general, patients who are neurologically intact do not aspirate even while sleeping. Chronic aspiration should be considered in patients who have mental retardation, recreational drug use or excessive alcohol consumption with a suggestive pattern of pneumonia.

IMMUNE FUNCTION STUDIES

The work-up of a patient with a suspected immune defect can be considered in two stages. The preliminary stage is a general evaluation. If this stage is normal, and HIV infection is not suspected, it is less likely that the patient has an immune defect. The pattern of infection should be used as a guide to specific investigations. Systemic viral infections

INVESTIGATION OF SUSPECTED IMMUNE DEFECTS

Preliminary Investigation

Complete blood count with differential

Platelets

Quantitative immunoglobulins

IgG subclasses

Secretory IgA

Specific antibodies

  Isohemagglutinins

  Immunized antigens

  Tetanus, diphtheria, mumps, and haemophilus

  Booster immunizations

Delayed cutaneous response

  Purified protein derivative (PPD) 50 TU/mL

  Candida 500 PNU/mL

  Trichophyton 1:30 dilution

  Tetanus toxoid 10 Lf/mL

  Mumps 40 cfu/mL

  Dinitrochlorobenzene (DNCB)

Laboratory Assessment of Immune Function

T-cell and B-cell studies

  Surface markers

  In vitro T-cell responses

MHC Class II

Note: If the preliminary investigation is suspicious, then a more specific immune work-up is indicated. See text for details.

and infections with unusual organisms suggest a cellular defect and a T-cell work-up. Recurrent abscess formation indicates the need for a work-up of polymorphonuclear (PMN) cell function (Table 13-1).

Preliminary Investigation

The initial work-up for a suspected immune defect consists of tests that have general applicability.

Complete Blood Count with Differential

The total number of cells and the number of lymphocytes and polymorphonuclear cells is helpful.

Low total lymphocyte numbers are seen in HIV infection and other T-cell disorders. Neutropenia can occur for many reasons including drug reactions and viruses. Low total white blood cell count is suggestive of aplastic anemia, drug reaction, or malignancy.

Patients who have a rare disorder of cyclic neutropenia present with recurrent infections on a monthly or 6 weekly basis. Serial complete blood counts will detect the fall in polymorphonuclear cells.

Platelets

Platelets are small and reduced in number in Wiskott-Aldrich syndrome. There may be thrombocytopenia as part of developmental anomalies with defects in immunity.

Quantitative Immunoglobulins

Total immunoglobulins can readily be measured in serum or plasma, using a variety of rapid and accurate techniques. The results are reported in mg/dL.

It is important to use age appropriate values for immunoglobulin levels in serum. At 1 year of age, the levels of IgG, IgM, and IgA are about 60% of adult values. An IgG level of 250–300 mg/dL is normal for a 3-month-old infant, but significantly reduced for an adult.

Significance. The immunoglobulin levels are an indication of general immune function. Low values are an indication for further work-up to delineate the source defect. By itself, a low immunoglobulin level does not indicate an immune defect. There may be low levels of IgG as part of a transient hypogammaglobulinemia picture in a newborn, and of little clinical significance. There may also be low immunoglobulin levels, but the protein that is present may be functioning antibody, in which case the patient may not have an immune defect as an explanation for recurrent infections. At the other end of the scale, immunoglobulins may be markedly elevated to 2000 mg/dL, but the patient can have early immune deficiency. The most common cause for this presentation is early AIDS. In this situation, B cells are being driven to produce antibody in response to the presence of antigen, but lack the guidance of CD4 T cells. As a result, they produce "nonsense" immunoglobulin that does not carry specific coding for the antigen in the Fab hypervariable region. There is thus no feedback to switch off B-cell function, and they continue proliferating. These patients will have lymphadenopathy. A second cause for high levels of immunoglobulin in the face of immune defect is multiple myeloma, where immunoglobulin levels are high, but are produced by malignant cells and do not have antibody function. For this reason, it is necessary to measure specific antibody production as well as total immunoglobulin.

IgG Subclasses

Of the four IgG subclasses, only IgG2 seems to have predictive value for recurrent infections when it is low or absent. The level must be considered in the total context of the patient and the type of infection that the patient has. Isolated IgG2 deficiency is associated with recurrent upper airway infections with pneumococcus and haemophilus infection. It is also associated with IgA deficiency.

Secretory IgA

It is possible to measure IgA in saliva and other secretions. The clinical relevance is not clear. Patients may have absent or low serum IgA, but secretory may be present. In this instance, it is not clear whether the patient actually has an immune defect, since IgA functions as a secretory antibody. If both are absent, the patient will be liable to develop infections. Rarely, serum IgA may be present, but secretory absent.

Specific Antibodies

There are several readily available specific antibodies that can be measured as an indication of antibody production, as opposed to immunoglobulin that may not be specific for an antigen.

Isohemagglutinins. These are the naturally occurring antibodies directed against the group A and group B red cell membrane markers. They are a measure of intrinsic specific antibody production and are normally present from 3 months of age. In patients who are blood group O, the anti-A and anti-B are IgG antibodies, while those who are group A or group B have the corresponding antibody (anti-B for group A and anti-A for group B) in the IgM isotype. For rare patients who are group AB, the test is not useful.

Immunized antigens. Serum levels of antibodies to tetanus, diphtheria, mumps, and haemophilus are useful. Since the question is whether the patient can sustain an immune response, only IgG antibodies are relevant. IgM will rise immediately postimmunization, but is not present long term. The significance of IgA serum antibodies is unclear, and there is no benefit to measuring specific IgA to these antigens.

If the levels are low or absent, the patient should receive booster immunizations. The assay is then repeated 2–3 weeks later to allow for a secondary response. This may particularly be needed in adults, where unboosted titers will be low because of normal decay of antibody production over time. A lack of response following a booster is strongly suggestive of an immune defect. There may also be a selected inability to respond to only one or two antigens, usually carbohydrate containing organisms, haemophilus and pneumococcus.

An abnormal or low response to specific antibody measurements is an indication for further work-up.

Delayed Cutaneous Response

The delayed cutaneous response is mediated by T cells interacting with macrophages. It is the mechanism for regulation of organisms such as *M. tuberculosis*. It is possible to test in vivo for this response, which is an important indicator of cellular immune function.

Antigens are injected intradermally or introduced by a prick into the dermis. The usual site is the anterior aspect of the forearm. A multitest device can be used, and is commercially available with T-cell antigens preloaded. Antigens that are used in this test include the following:

- Purified protein derivative (PPD) 50 TU/mL
- Candida 500 PNU/mL
- Trichophyton 1:30 dilution

- Tetanus toxoid 10 Lf/mL
- Mumps 40 cfu/mL

Controls consist of the vehicle used to dissolve the antigens, usually saline.

The test is read after 48 hours. A positive test is a weal reaction, usually –10 mm in diameter. Most people should be positive to Candida and Trichophyton and mumps, and these antigens are often used as positive controls when doing a PPD test to diagnose possible tuberculosis.

If there is no response to these antigens, further work-up is indicated.

Dinitrochlorobenzene (DNCB). In patients who do not respond to delayed response antigens, it is possible to challenge with agents that induce a strong T-cell response. DNCB and keyhole limpet hemocyanin are potent agents that stimulate T-cell responses in vivo and in vitro. They are not approved for clinical use, and should only be applied by physicians familiar with the use of these agents, as they can cause painful skin lesions and possible systemic effects.

The technique involves painting DNCB onto an area of the forearm or upper arm and applying an occlusive dressing for 24 hours. The site is evaluated for sensitization in 10–14 days. A challenge dose is then applied to the opposite arm to assess systemic response. This dose is usually 5% of the sensitizing dose. If the patient has responded, they will develop a lesion in 12–24 hours at the challenge site. The lesion is erythematous, indurated, and perhaps vesicular. Biopsy shows spongiosus with variable epidermal degeneration and macrophage and DR+/CD3+ lymphocytic infiltration

There is not always a clinical correlation between the response to DNCB and clinical T-cell function. These responses should be confirmed by in vitro tests.

Laboratory Assessment of Immune Function

T-Cell and B-Cell Studies

The investigation of lymphoytes involves delineating the surface markers and proliferative function.

T cells. An evaluation of immune function will include assessment of the distribution of T-cell subclasses. This is performed by allowing the cells to react with antibodies to the surface structures of lymphocytes known as cluster of differentiation (CD) markers. The antibodies have an attached fluorescent marker (usually fluorescein or rhodamine). The stained cells are passed through a flow cytometer and the percentage of cells that react with each marker is noted as a percentage of the whole.

There are three key CD markers that identify groups of T cells. Function does not correlate well with surface markers. The major markers are shown in Table 13-2.

Surface markers

CD3: The universal T-cell marker is CD3. Its presence on the cell indicates that it is a mature T cell. It also takes part in almost all immune reactions involving T cells. Absence or a low level of cells that are CD3+ indicates a severe immune defect (Table 13-2).

CD4: This population of T cells (CD3+4+8–) constitutes two-thirds of the CD3 positive population. The presence of this marker also denotes a mature cell. Helper function has been found among this population of T cells, but it is probably not correct to term them helper cells, as they are responsible for a wide range of functions. This population also carries a receptor for the Fc component of IgM.

TABLE 13-2

MAJOR T-CELL MARKERS THAT ARE INVOLVED IN T-CELL RECOGNITION

T Cell Subset	Function
CD3	All T cells
CD4	Helper cells
CD8	Suppressor cells
CD56	Natural killer cells
CD11b	Adhesion
T receptor	All T cells
CD1a	Thymocytes

Note: Function is only loosely correlated with surface markes.

Absence or a low level of these cells is seen in a number of cellular immune defects. In AIDS this subset of T cells is selectively destroyed, leading to severe immune deficiencies. In some forms of Ebstein-Barr virus infection, a similar pattern can be found, with low CD3+4+8– cells.

CD8: The CD8 subset of T cells (CD3+4–8+) is also a mature population of cells. While suppressor function is attributed to these cells, they are not completely understood.

Low levels or absence of these cells is found in severe combined immune defects and in isolated T-cell deficiencies such as Di George syndrome.

CD4/CD8: This is a useful ratio, which is normally 1.5–2:1. It is altered in AIDS and may be low in some congenital immune defects. An abnormal ratio indicates a serious abnormality of immune function.

CD1a: This is a primitive thymocyte marker, along with CD1b and CD1c. It is not normally found beyond embryogenesis, and is diagnostic of a lack of thymic function during development.

CD56: This ligand has several different functions on various cell types. On T cells it is associated with natural killer activity. These are cells with potent antiviral properties.

They may be present even in thymic deficiency.

Common

MHC Class II: The MHC Class II is a measure of immune cell activation. It will be expressed strongly on B cells in early AIDS even in the face of falling CD4 cells.

CD11b: This marker is an integrin molecule and is an important ligand for endothelial adhesion molecules. It is found on polymorphonuclear cells where it has an important function in leukocyte adherence and in ingesting opsonized antigens. CD11b is absent in leukocyte adhesion deficiency. It is also present on all mononuclear cells

In vitro T-cell responses.

T-cell proliferative studies are difficult to perform, and are often done in immunology research laboratories.

Method: Extraction of lymphocytes: The patient's peripheral blood is fractionated over a density gradient of Ficoll-Hypaque and the lymphocyte layer is removed. After washing, the cells are placed into microtiter wells in culture medium. The test antigen is added and 10^5 cells/well cultured at 37°C in 5% CO_2 for 3–5 days. Radiolabeled thymidine is added and the culture is continued overnight. The cells are harvested onto filter discs, being lysed with water. Radiolabeled DNA adheres to the filter discs, which are placed into counting wells with beta radiation counting fluid. DNA proliferation is inferred from counts of radiation. The result is usually expressed as stimulation index (SI), which compares the cells with and without antigen. Background counts are subtracted, so that the SI of the control is zero.

Antigens: There are two groups of antigens, mitogens and antigens. Mitogens are potent antigens that are usually derived from plants. They stimulate nearly all T cells to divide. On the other hand, antigens such as tetanus only stimulate approximately 10% of T cells to divide.

The usual mitogens are the following:

- Phytohemagglutinin (PHA)
- Concanavalin A (Con A)
- Pokeweed mitogen (PWM)

There are a limited number of antigens that are commonly used. Commercial availability of antigens in a form suitable for in vitro testing is limited. Candida and Trichophyton are used. Tetanus toxoid is no longer available. Other antigens are used if they are purified as part of a research protocol.

Heterologous lymphocytes may be placed in culture using a technique called mixed leukocyte reaction to assess whether they will react to each other. This is important in bone marrow transplant. One set of lymphocytes may be irradiated or treated with mitomycin to prevent cell division so only one set is tested at a time.

A clinical example is given in Table 13-3.

EXAMPLE OF LYMPHOPROLIFERATIVE STUDIES FROM A PATIENT WITH A T-CELL DEFECT

Antigen	SI Control	SI Patient
PHA	260	10
Con A	110	15
PWM	96	5
Candida	20	0
Tetanus toxoid	25	0
MLR patient irradiated	30	0
MLR control irradiated	0	0

Note: Equal numbers of cells are studied in control and patient, so differences are due to lymphocyte responses. There is a marked reduction in response of the patient's lymphocytes. In the MLR, the patient does not respond to control cells, but the control responds well to patient's lymphocytes. SI: stimulation index; PHA: phytohemagglutinin; Con A: concanavalin A; PWM: Pokeweed mitogen; MLR: mixed leukocyte reaction.

B cells. An assessment of B-cell subclasses is in Table 13–4.

Surface markers

Immunoglobulins: B cells have their own set of surface markers. They are further distinct from T cells in that they have immunoglobulin on their surface and in cytoplasm. There is a high concentration of IgD with a lower level of IgM. There is

TYPICAL B-CELL MARKERS DETECTED BY FLOW CYTOMETRY

B Cell Subset	Function
CD-9	Pre-B-cells
CD-19	B cells
CD-5	B Cell
CD-21	Complement
CDw32	Fc receptor
Anti-IgD	Immunoglobulin
Anti-IgM	Immunoglobulin

also intracytoplasmic immunoglobulin. In patients with Bruton's agammaglobulinemia, only intracytoplasmic immunoglobulin is present, indicating that only primitive cells are present.

CD19: This marker appears early in embryogenesis and persists as a B-cell marker.

CD9: This is an embryonic marker that usually is not present on mature B cells.

CD5: This surface structure appears during embryogenesis and persists. It seems to be connected to the development of tolerance.

CD21: This is one of the receptors for complement on the B-cell surface that serves an important function.

CDw32: The Fc receptor is very important. Immunoglobulin binds to B cells by this receptor. B cells also retain immunoglobulin that they make on the cell surface.

Functional studies. Functional studies of B cells derived from peripheral blood are not commercially available. The B cells that seem to respond are in the secondary immune organs, the lymph nodes, spleen, tonsil, and bone marrow. B cells in circulation do not respond to stimulation in vitro and it is difficult to induce them to produce antibody.

Polymorphonuclear (PMN) Function

The function of PMNs falls into three categories: migration and adhesion, phagocytosis, and killing.

Migration. Tests that assess the response of PMN to chemotactic stimuli use common techniques. A Boyden chamber is a two chambered device, with a semipermeable membrane separating them. A suspension of white cells is placed in one chamber, and a chemoattractant agent in the other. After incubation, the membrane is removed, stained with a white cell stain and the number of PMNs adherent to the membrane is counted. The results for the patient are compared to a normal control.

Adhesion. A large number of adhesion molecules have been described on endothelium and other cells. Examples include the selectin family, which is important for binding to activated endothelium

TABLE 13-5

OVERALL SUMMARY OF INVESTIGATIONS FOR IMMUNE FUNCTION AND HOW THEY APPLY TO SPECIFIC CELL TYPES

	T Cells	B Cells	Neutrophils	Macrophages
Surface markers	CD	CD	CD	CD
Proliferation	++++	+	–	–
Killing	++	–	++++	+++
Mediator production	++++	+	+++	++++
Antibody production	–	++++[a]	–	–
Phagocytosis	–	–	++++	++++
O_2^- production	–	–	++++	+++
MHC Class II expression	With activation	With activation	With activation	With activation

[a]Peripheral blood B cells do not readily make antibodies in vitro. + = has this function.

and lymphocyte homing. The integrin family is a collection of heterodimers that function as ligands in a number of cell functions. The immunoglobulin gene superfamily is an important group of adhesion molecules. These molecules are detected by specific staining, both in situ and by flow cytometry. Abnormalities of adhesion molecules have been described that cause recurrent bacterial infections and inadequate PMN function.

Phagocytosis and killing. It is difficult to separate these functions, as they are interdependent.

Ingestion of organisms can be measured directly, using opsonized staphylococcus and counting the percentage of organism ingested. Indirect measurement can be made using a stimulant of the respiratory burst such as phorbol myristate (PMA), and measuring superoxide production. In conditions such as chronic granulomatous disease, the response to PMA is blunted. An older test, the nitroblue tetrazolium (NBT) slide test is convenient, but its accuracy has been questioned. It is an indirect measure of superoxide production. NBT is a soluble yellow dye that is reduced by superoxide to formazan, an insoluble precipitate that stains the cells dark blue or black. In normal patients, almost all the PMNs on a slide will show dark granules, while in patients with CGD, the cells will remain unstained.

Complement

Total complement function can be detected by lysis of mouse red blood cells. The endpoint of the assay is the lysis of 50% of the cells, and the result is expressed as total hemolytic complement in units or as CH50.

Assays are available for all of the components of complement, which can be specifically measured if a patient is suspected of being deficient in a complement component.

Table 13-5 provides an overview of immune cells and the functions that can be assessed in vitro.

Intrauterine Diagnosis and Carrier Detection

Newer technologies of intrauterine diagnosis make it possible to detect ADA and PNP deficiencies by enzyme analyses on cells from amniotic fluid. Using restriction fragment length polymorphism several X-linked defects including SCID or other severe T-cell deficiencies, CGD, or Wiskott-Aldrich syndrome can be diagnosed. In the case of those disorders for which the defective gene has been cloned and cDNA probes are available, the diagnosis can be made by deletional or RFLP analyses of chorionic villus samples obtained during the first trimester.

Part II. Therapy

OVERALL THERAPY

Where possible, the underlying disease should be identified. Treatment of the basic disease is specific for this problem. For example, a sequestered lung lobe will require surgical correction, as will vascular anomalies obstructing a bronchus. Bronchoscopy may be needed to remove a foreign body lodged in a bronchus. In cases where the immune defect is secondary to an autoimmune disease or malignancy, the focus of therapy is the primary condition.

MANAGEMENT OF THE INFECTION

Antibiotics

Immediate

Controlling the infection in immunodeficient diseases is the primary problem. Infection is often by resistant or unusual organisms. Cultures should be obtained where possible and appropriate antibiotics used. Depending on the type of immune defect, some assumptions can be made. In CGD, for example, the most likely organism is *staphylococcus* or *serratia* sp., and therapy can be started with a drug that might give appropriate coverage.

Long Term

Maintaining patients with an immune defect free of infection is difficult. If prophylactic antibiotics are used, they should be rotated every 3 months. A prophylactic dose is usually given daily. If a resistant organism emerges, the antibiotic regimen should be changed accordingly.

Prophylactic Antimicrobials

The use of antibiotics to prevent infections is often successful, especially if the infections predominantly occur in the upper airway. An approach might be to administer Bactrim daily for 3 months, then change to Ceclor 250–500 mg daily for 3

months followed by amoxicillin, 250–500 mg daily and restarting the course.

Adjunctive Measures

Any cause of stasis or accumulation of secretions should be treated aggressively. Approaches to remove secretions include chest physical therapy and bronchoscopy.

Chest Physical Therapy

Frequent chest physical therapy is helpful in preventing bronchiectasis. New forms of administering this therapy at home, such as the Vest are very efficient and provide a considerable improvement over hand percussion for chest physical therapy. One schedule is to use the Vest for 20 minutes twice per day. Another useful group of devices uses an oscillatory principle to generate a shear force along the bronchi to loosen mucus. One such device is the Flutter, which looks like a pipe with a ball in the bowl. As the patient exhales, the ball vibrates, sending a wave front into the bronchi that creates a shear force along the walls, loosening mucus.

A useful technique that has been used in cystic fibrosis and in patients who have bronchiectasis, is the Huff breathing method. In this method, the patient takes a slow deep breath using diaphragmatic breathing in an attempt to build pressure behind the mucus. Building up a volume of air behind the mucus helps to propel it toward the mouth. The patient pauses, and then coughs twice with the mouth slightly open. The patient pauses again and then inhales by sniffing gently. Taking in a big breath after coughing may drive the mucus back into the lungs.

Bronchoscopy

There are two methods of performing this procedure, rigid and fiberoptic. The easier method is by a fibrescope. For bronchoscopy, this has one or two additional channels, depending on the size. In small units, for children, there is often only one channel. The advantage of the fiberoptic unit is that it can be used without anesthetic, and only sedation and local anesthetic are required. This scope can be used for identification of intrabronchial conditions, suctioning and collecting samples for precise bacteriologic or virologic diagnosis. Bronchoscopy is the most reliable method of detecting organisms such as Pneumocystis, as sputum collection often fails to detect the organism. It is also possible to take biopsies by this method. These are usually transbronchial, and are most useful for detecting malignancies that arise in the bronchi, and less useful for parenchymal disease.

The fiberoptic method is limited in small children who need supplemental oxygen because there is only one channel, so the patient cannot receive O_2 and be suctioned at the same time. This type of scope does not allow for the removal of foreign objects from the bronchi, which is a significant limitation in the case of a patient who has a pattern of infection that suggests that there might be a foreign body present.

Rigid bronchoscopy is performed with a metal tube that has an open lumen. The patient must be anesthetized for the procedure. This type of bronchoscope has the advantage that procedures such as the removal of a foreign body can easily be accomplished. Suctioning is safer as it is easier to give O_2 to a potentially unstable patient. Having to use an anesthetic is a drawback of the procedure.

TREAT UNDERLYING CONDITIONS

Aspiration

A key to managing recurrent infections is controlling any underlying conditions. Patients who are mentally impaired have a high risk of recurrent aspiration of food or saliva. This carries a serious danger of severe pneumonia with anaerobic organisms. Patients in this state should be fed by gastrostomy tube, and, if gastroesophageal reflux is present, an antireflux procedure should be performed.

Heart Disease

Underlying congenital heart defects can be corrected where possible. Causes of venous pulmonary congestion should be controlled.

Relieve Obstruction

Where feasible, obstructions to hollow organs by a mass, foreign body, or swelling should be resolved. Examples are shown in Table 13-6.

AVOID HIGH RISK SITUATIONS

Sources of Infection

In the normal course, growing children are exposed to numerous situations that increase their risk of developing infections. Day care centers, nursery schools, school and play centers are concentrations of viruses and bacteria that children share. These exposures are useful in the development of a library of immune cells that can respond to a variety of antigens. For a child with an immune defect, this type of exposure can be disastrous. This risk is compounded by the common problem that children with immune defects are not immunized because they are frequently ill. Even if they receive immunizations, their response is poor and they will often not have protective levels of antibody. As a result, there is a significant risk to a child with an immune defect attending nursery schools and day care centers.

Children with immune defects should be advised to avoid these high risk situations and should not be placed in nursery school. Caution should also be exerted for birthday parties and being around people with infections, even if they seem innocuous. Adults with immune defects should avoid others with infections and be careful around children, who are frequent carriers of viral and other infections.

Blood Products

Plasma

If patients have an IgA deficiency and receive a blood transfusion, or whole plasma, their immune system

TABLE 13-6

COMMON MECHANICAL PROBLEMS THAT LEAD TO RECURRENT INFECTIONS, AND SOLUTIONS TO PREVENT THE RECURRENT INFECTIONS

Problem	Solution
Foreign object in the airway causing recurrent infections distal to the obstruction	Removal by bronchoscopy
Anatomic abnormalities of the sinus cavity leading to infection	Prophylactic antibiotics Surgical correction
Eustachian tube dysfunction, common in childhood and upper airway allergies, leading to recurrent otitis media	Antibiotic therapy Tympanostomy tube placement
Posterior urethral valves causing stasis of urine and recurrent urinary tract infections in male infants	Immediate bladder catheterization Surgical correction
Sequestrated lobe of the lung, with poor gas exchange and air stasis, that leads to chronic and recurrent pneumonia	Surgical removal of the infected lobe
Bronchiectasis	Prophylactic antibiotics Chest physical therapy Surgical removal of the bronchiectatic segments
Loculated infection, for example, empyema	Surgical drainage

will interpret the IgA as a foreign protein and make antibodies, resulting in immune response that produces IgG that is anti-IgA. This effectively removes the infused IgA, and can lead to the formation of circulating immune complexes with vasculitis.

Cells

There is a significant problem attendant on infusing viable lymphocytes and monocytes into a patient who is immunocompromised. A condition arises that is known as graft v. host disease (GVHD). This same condition arises as a complication of bone marrow transplantation, and is discussed below.

Type of Blood Products to Use

In patients with immune defects who need a blood transfusion, only packed, washed and irradiated red cells should be infused. Washing the cells removes any immunoglobulin or other strongly antigenic proteins that might be adsorbed onto the cell, and reduces the risk of a severe reaction. Irradiating the blood damages and cross-links the DNA of lympho-

cytes, preventing them from dividing and activating. Since GVHD is caused by T cells, irradiating will prevent this complication.

Vaccines

The administration of vaccines presents a problem in children with immune defects, particularly if there is reduced or absent T-cell function and numbers. No live virus vaccines should be given since there is a risk of causing disseminated infection that may be fatal. Even with killed virus vaccines, the patient will not make antibodies in response to an injection. For this reason, it is important for parents to be aware when other children are ill and avoid contact with the sick child.

REPLACEMENT THERAPIES

Gamma Globulin Replacement

In selected patients, it is possible to replace the missing or malfunctioning gamma globulin.

Specifically, only IgG is available for replacement. This form therapy helps to control infections in patients with hypogammaglobulinemias. Only patients who have IgG deficiency will benefit from this treatment. It is not indicated for IgA or IgM deficiency.

Dose

Replacement doses of gamma globulin are based on 400 mg/kg. The dose is given intravenously every 3–4 weeks. The intravenous infusion is started slowly and the rate gradually increased to avoid side effects. Side effects may include fever, rash, hypotension, and arthralgia.

Enzyme Replacement

Several attempts have been made to correct immune deficiencies by replacing absent or defective enzymes. Adenosine deaminase deficiency has shown partial improvement in response to red cell infusion. This effect does not persist. To date, sustaining the effect remains a problem, and for this reason, enzyme replacement has limited clinical use.

Gene Replacement

Although some benefits have been shown with gene replacement therapy, there is still much that is unknown about the functions of genes. Recently, a group of SCID patients received gene-corrected autologous bone marrow transplants. Of the eleven patients, nine acquired normal immune function. As of this writing, two patients have developed a leukemia-like syndrome, which responded to chemotherapy. Much seems promising about the future of gene therapy research, but the science is still in its infancy stages.

TRANSPLANT

Bone Marrow

Bone marrow transplantation can potentially restore immune competence in patients who have severe immune defects.

Technique

The ideal donor for bone marrow would be an identical twin. The most important feature that distinguishes bone marrow from other organs is that bone marrow is strongly immunocompetent tissue. For this reason, it is important to obtain as close a match as possible between the donor and the patient. The key sites of discrepancy that can cause either rejection of the graft, or graft v. host disease are the MHC complex (Classes I and II) and the ABO blood type. The first choice is for a donor who is identical, either related or unrelated to the patient.

Graft v. Host disease (GVHD)

This is a condition that is the result of infusing competent lymphocytes into an immune incompetent host. The result is that the infused cells react to the host MHC and proceed to reject the host, often with a fatal outcome. The incidence and severity of GVHD correlates directly with the degree of major histocompatability complex mismatch. However, even among recipients of MHC antigen–identical marrows, 40% develop acute GVHD. With only one antigen mismatch, the frequency rise to 60–80% who develop acute GVHD. Children are more resistant to developing GVHD than adults. Both allogeneic (between two individuals) and autologous (from the same individual) grafts cause GVHD.

Pathophysiology. The mechanism of development of GVHD is shown in Figure 13-1.

The criteria described by Billingham in 1966 still apply to the development of GVHD. In general, the graft must contain immunologically competent cells, the host must appear foreign to the graft, and the host must be immunocompromised and incapable of reacting against the graft. While the extent of histoincompatibility between donor and host and the residual number of T cells in the graft have a major impact on the incidence of GVHD, even autologous grafts show GVHD. In the instance of autologous grafts, the recipient is usually receiving cyclosporine.

The initiation of GVHD involves recognition of epithelial target tissues of the host as foreign by the transplanted immunocompetent cells. This results

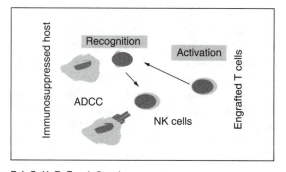

FIGURE 13-1

REPRESENTATION OF THE MECHANISM OF GVHD.

Immunocompetent immune cells are infused into an immunosuppressed or immune deficient host. The infused cells become engrafted into the host. Surface tissue MHC is recognized as foreign by the engrafted cells, which then react and cause tissue destruction within the host.

in immune activation of these cells with subsequent induction of an inflammatory response and death of the target tissue. T cells mainly orchestrate the initial inflammatory response. Subsequently, many cell types including CD4+, CD8+, and natural killer cells are found at sites of tissue injury.

Increases in serum IgE levels from sevenfold to 2000-fold have been reported in patients after bone marrow transplantation. This rise is thought to be due to soluble CD23 product that is a fragment of the low-affinity IgE receptor.

Clinical features of GVHD

Age risk:

Younger than 20 years—20% risk
45–50 years—30% risk
Older than 50 years—80% risk

Staging: There are four stages of acute GVHD, which are described in Table 13-7. The staging depends on the degree and severity of skin involvement. Mortality increases from stage 1 to 4.

Acute: GVHD occurs within the first 100 days of a transplant. It typically causes dermatitis, enteritis, and hepatitis.

Initial lesions are scattered erythematous macules and papules that spread as the disease increases. Erythroderma and bullae are the most severe form of the disease.

TABLE 13-7

STAGING OF ACUTE GVHD

Stage	Features
1	<25% body surface involvement
2	25–50% body surface involvement
3	50–100% body surface involvement
4	Vesicles and bullae

Note: The course can be fulminant or arrest at any stage.

Eruptions usually begin as faint tender erythematous macules on any body part (palms and soles often present first) and often form preferentially around the hair follicle. As the disease progresses, the lesions coalesce and form confluent erythema. Papules emerge at this stage. The most severe form is the subepidermal bullous form. At this stage the disease resembles toxic epidermal necrolysis.

Chronic: Patients enter this phase after day 100. In essence, this is an autoimmune syndrome directed toward multiple organs. The skin is the primary organ involved in chronic GVHD, which can manifest as a lichen planus–like or scleroderma–like eruptions.

The risk of developing chronic GVHD increases with the severity of acute GVHD, and patients with stage 3 or stage 4 acute disease are more likely to progress to chronic stages than patients with stage 1 or stage 2 acute disease. Progression of the skin disease is to violaceous lichenified papules that are indistinguishable from lichen planus and occur on flexor surfaces. There can be further progression to sclerodermatous changes.

Systemic involvement included the GI tract, with chronic diarrhea and weight loss. Hepatic involvement is often a major contributor to mortality, with chronic liver failure developing in a high percentage of patients. Joint involvement can lead to contractures. The patients are very susceptible to sepsis and other infections, which are a significant cause for mortality.

Mortality. GVHD is a significant cause for death in marrow transplantation. Patients with acute GVHD are at risk for sepsis, electrolyte disturbances secondary to diarrhea, elevated liver enzyme levels, bilirubinemia, and hepatorenal syndrome. In chronic GVHD, patients develop joint contractures, ulceration, esophageal strictures, keratoconjunctivitis sicca, and global immune impairment. Death occurs in 15–40% of patients in the acute phase of GVHD, and in a high percentage of those with chronic disease. The more severe and extensive the involvement, the greater is the risk of mortality. Overwhelming sepsis is the primary cause of death.

Differential. The differential diagnosis will vary with the stage of the disease and the conditions the GVHD may resemble. These include the following:

- Contact dermatis
- Drug eruptions
- Erythroderma
- Lichen planus
- Staphylococcal scalded skin syndrome
- Stevens-Johnson syndrome
- Toxic epidermal necrolysis
- Toxic shock syndrome

Modification to transplant material. In an attempt to reduce the risk of GVHD, various manipulations have been used on the donor marrow prior to transplantation. The most widely used are techniques that remove T cells from the marrow. The idea is that by allowing the T cells to reform from precursors, they will not recognize the host as foreign. This manipulation has not prevented GVHD from occurring.

Thymus

Thymic epithelial tissue has been used to induce the emergence of immunocompetent T cells. This technique has been used particularly in patients with Di George syndrome and other forms of thymic hypoplasia.

The technique involves using allogeneic postnatal cultured thymus tissue. Thinly sliced thymic tissue is inserted extraperitoneally. Newer experimental procedures may connect directly to the vasculature. Using this method, a recent study demonstrated that 7 of 12 patients with Di George syndrome had survived long term. They demonstrated increased T-cell proliferation and immune competence. Most of the immune competence recovery occurred in 1 year posttransplant. Ideally, transplantation should occur before the patients develop infections. The technique is being studied in combination with retroviral agents for control of HIV infection.

The risks and complications include the following:

- Cytomegalovirus infection
- Eosinophilia
- Rash
- Lymphadenopathy
- Development of CD4–CD8–(primitive) peripheral T cells
- Elevated serum immunoglobulin E (IgE)
- Possible pulmonary inflammation
- Lymphoma has been reported

STEM CELL TRANSPLANTATION

Sources for stem cells include bone marrow and umbilical cord blood. Undifferentiated fetal cells also have the potential for such use. Further, stem cells can be derived from bone marrow of an MHC-identical sibling or haploidentical parent or relative. Cells can also be derived from bone marrow or blood of a matched, unrelated donor. As for bone marrow, T cells may also be removed from the stem cell preparation.

Theoretically, the use of stem cells carries a lower risk of GVHD, and can result in more rapid reconstitution of bone marrow. This advantage probably relates to the totipotent nature of stem cells.

Suggested Reading

Barker, J. N. and J. E. Wagner (2003). Umbilical-cord blood transplantation for the treatment of cancer. *Nat Rev Cancer* **3**(7): 526–32.

Dean, R. M. and M. R. Bishop (2003). Graft-versus-host disease: emerging concepts in prevention and therapy. *Curr Hematol Rep* **2**(4): 287–94.

Dizon, J. G., B. J. Goldberg, et al. (1998). How to evaluate suspected immunodeficiency [comment]. *Pediatr Ann* **27**(11): 743–50.

Folds, J. D. and J. L. Schmitz (2003). 24. Clinical and laboratory assessment of immunity. *J Allergy Clin Immunol* **111**(2 Suppl): S702–11.

Horwitz, M. E. (2000). Stem-cell transplantation for inherited immunodeficiency disorders. *Pediatr Clin North Am* **47**(6): 1371–87.

Knezevic-Maramica, I. and M. S. Kruskall (2003). Intravenous immune globulins: an update for clinicians. *Transfusion* **43**(10): 1460–80.

Maloney, D. G., B. M. Sandmaier, et al. (2002). Nonmyeloablative transplantation. *Hematology*: 392–421.

Noroski, L. M. and W. T. Shearer (1998). Screening for primary immunodeficiencies in the clinical immunology laboratory. *Clin Immunol Immunopathol* **86**(3): 237–45.

Paul, M. E. (2002). Diagnosis of immunodeficiency: clinical clues and diagnostic tests. *Curr Allergy Asthma Rep* **2**(5): 349–55.

Reddy, P. and J. L. Ferrara (2003). Role of interleukin-18 in acute graft-vs-host disease. *J Lab Clin Med* **141**(6): 365–71.

Rodriguez, T. E. and P. J. Stiff (2003). Current treatment results of allogeneic bone marrow transplantation for acute myeloid and lymphoid leukemia. *Curr Hematol Rep* **2**(4): 295–301.

Schwartz, S. A. (2000). Intravenous immunoglobulin treatment of immunodeficiency disorders. *Pediatr Clin North Am* **47**(6): 1355–69.

Tangsinmankong, N., S. L. Bahna, et al. (2001). The immunologic workup of the child suspected of immunodeficiency. *Ann Allergy Asthma Immunol* **87**(5): 362–9; quiz 370, 423.

Wingard, J. R., G. B. Vogelsang, et al. (2002). Stem cell transplantation: supportive care and long-term complications. *Hematology*: 422–44

14

MEDICATIONS AND THERAPEUTIC METHODS

There is considerable overlap among the medications that are used for allergies and asthma. Delivery of these medications is not simple, resulting in a proliferation of devices to dispense doses of medication to the patient. There is a need to educate the patient (and parents in the case of a child) in the use of these devices. The techniques for using these dispensers are not always easy or self-evident, and teaching their use should be built into the care plan. Revision is needed at each visit. Patients often have poor use of devices and discontinue the use of medication because of the complexity of using these dispensers. This chapter reviews available devices and medications in common use for allergies and asthma.

DEVICES FOR ASTHMA

There are a number of devices that are used to dispense inhaled asthma medications. All require that the patient have instruction in their use, with frequent review of technique. Most are easily used incorrectly, resulting in poor delivery of medication. The purpose of these devices is to deliver medication to the lower airway. The ideal device will

- Have a high concentration of particles in the size range of 3–5 μm which is ideal for deposition on the airway mucosa of medium size bronchi
- Disperse in a controlled manner, allowing time for inhalation
- Have uniform dose measurement
- There are three basic modes of delivery
  - Metered Dose Inhalation (MDI)
  - Dry Powder Inhalation (DPI)
  - Nebulizer

Metered Dose Inhaler (MDI)

Structure

This type of device is a double chambered cylinder. There is a larger pressurized chamber which acts as a reservoir holding the medication. The second is a small metering valve that acts as a holding chamber to contain the next dose of medication. The device is placed in a plastic actuator that is molded with a mouthpiece. The canister and plastic sleeve are engineered for different types of propellant, and are not interchangeable.

The typical design is shown in Figure 14-1.

The medication in this device is in the form of a microfine powder that is suspended in a gaseous

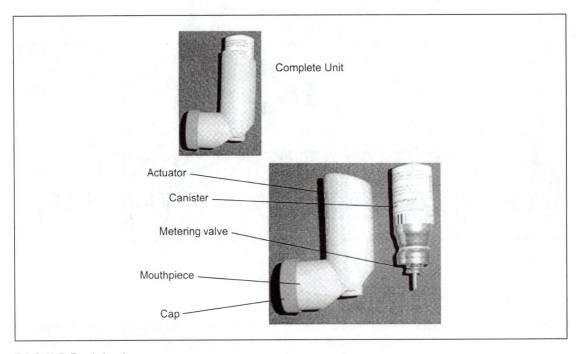

FIGURE 14-1

COMPONENTS OF A METERED DOSE INHALER.

propellant. Chlorofluorocarbon (CFC) was the usual propellant, and has been discontinued completely as of 2003 as part of a worldwide effort to eliminate this chemical because of its damaging effect on the atmospheric ozone layer. It also had the problem of being temperature dependent and having an unpleasant taste. Because CFCs expand rapidly, the nozzle speed is high with these devices, making inhalation difficult. Tetrafluoroethane (HFA13a) is one replacement propellant that has gained popularity. It has a sweetish taste and a much lower nozzle speed than CFCs. The smaller holding chamber is filled from the canister and holds a precisely measured dose of the drug. When the canister is depressed from the top, the drug in the holding chamber is released in a pear shaped cloud. With HFA13a, the dispersion pattern is softer, and leaves the nozzle with less force.

This is a gravity-feed device, and needs to be right side up. The patient must be sure to prime a new unit. The canister should be well shaken before each use, as the powder settles. The patient should always use more than one inhalation, and dosing should be adjusted accordingly. This corrects the frequent problem of leakage from the metering valve while the device is unused. Thus, the first dose may deliver less than the metered amount.

The MDI canisters can be evaluated for the amount of medication that remains by placing them (without plastic holder) in a bowl of water and observe whether they float horizontally at the top (empty), sink to the bottom (full), or float halfway between top and bottom (half-full). This method only works for CFC propelled devices. Most MDIs hold 200 doses.

MDI Techniques

General principles

- Education should be done in the office during the visit when patients start on an inhaler.

- Checks of technique should occur during follow-up visits. The use of MDIs is extremely technique dependent, and frequent revision is essential.
- It is useful to use samples in the office, or placebo inhalers for demonstration. Actually have the patient take a dose in the office in front of the person explaining the technique.
- Give feedback immediately and correct bad technique. Ask the patient to demonstrate the technique.
- Give written instructions for the patient to take home.
- Having the pharmacy give the patient instructions is often reinforcing, but the set-up in most pharmacies is not conducive to learning the proper use of an MDI.

There are two techniques for using an MDI without a spacer—open mouth and closed mouth.

Closed-mouth technique

- Hold the canister upright and shake the MDI. Remove the cap.
- The patient should stand in a relaxed manner.
- It is important that the MDI be placed between the teeth and the tongue positioned underneath the inhaler opening out of the way.
- The patient should initiate a steady breath. After about 10% of the breath is inhaled, he/she should actuate the canister. Inhalation should be at a steady pace. The patient should be told to hold their breath at the top of inhalation for 10 seconds, and then to breath out through their nose.
- After the first inhalation, have the patient wait for a few seconds, and then repeat.

Open-mouth technique

- Hold MDI two fingers width from wide-open mouth and direct toward the mouth. Use the fingers as a guide for correct positioning.
- Make sure mouth is wide open.
- Start a slow inhalation and actuate the MDI at the same time. Complete the inhalation as noted for closed-mouth technique.
- The use of a spacer device is simpler to master but may not be well accepted by all patients, especially teenagers.

Variant—maxair autohaler

- This device contains a standard canister holding pirbuterol, which is almost identical to albuterol. The propellant is CFC, and will be revised because of the ban on CFC. In place of the actuator, the canister is placed in an enclosed plastic container with a spring loaded lever at the top. There is a flap-valve at the mouthpiece that is pressure activated and fires automatically on inspiration. The advantage of this system is that it eliminates the complicated coordination of inhalation and activation that MDI use requires. The canister unit holds 400 doses. Since a spacer device is not needed, this is a useful delivery method for teenagers who may not have good MDI technique and are unlikely to use a spacer.
- The device is primed by lifting the lever at the top and shaking the canister. The Autohaler should be placed in the mouth with the same precautions as for a standard MDI. The patient should be instructed to inhale steadily and continue to full inhalation after a click is heard. The lever must be cocked again for the second dose. Because of the design of the mouthpiece, the puff is much softer than the usual MDI. A sharp, acrid taste indicates that the device was not adequately shaken and is due to undiluted propellant.

Common errors with MDIs

- Mist coming up through the canister (the *chimney sign*) usually means obstruction by the tongue or teeth. This problem will also occur if inhalation occurs too late after activation or the patient actually exhales after activating the canister.
- Mist coming out of the patient's mouth usually means that the patient did not inhale adequately after activation.
- The patient may activate too early/late during inhalation, or inhale too quickly or slowly.
- Breathing through the nose instead of the MDI.
- Inadequate inspiration or incomplete breath-holding.

Spacer Devices

Techniques for correct use of MDIs are difficult and they are seldom used properly or consistently. A spacer simplifies the administration of medication, and makes it easier and more efficient to use a pressurized spray device. It also extends the age at which MDIs can be used to small children.

Other advantages include the following:

- Slows down aerosol particle speed before entering the mouth.
- Decreases amount of medication impacting on oropharynx which is then swallowed.
- Helps patients use an MDI irrespective of age. Even young children can use the device with a modification of technique.
- Can help the patient maintain an optimal inspiratory rate without the timing difficulties inherent in either open- or closed-mouth technique.
- Reduces "bad taste" of medication.
- Collapsible spacers (InspirEase, EZ Spacer) provide a visual indication of the effectiveness of the patient's effort.
- Delivery of medication below the glottis is about 10–15%, which is the same as good MDI technique.

Spacer Design

A true spacer is a holding chamber with a one-way valve. This allows time for inhaling the medication delivered from an MDI. Moreover, the patient can take multiple breaths from each actuation to improve delivery below the glottis. The ideal spacer holds 750 mL and is pear shaped. This structure allows the plume from the MDI room to expand and remain in suspension with minimal rain-out on the walls of the chamber. Smaller devices (under 250 mL) are less successful. From a practical point of view, most devices are cylindrical, rather than pear shaped. Pear shaped devices are harder to carry and store, and are clumsier to use than cylinders or collapsible bags.

Examples are the following:

- InspirEase (collapsible bag)
- EZ Spacer (collapsible bag)
- Aerochamber (also available with mask) (cylinder)

- Optichamber (also available with mask) (cylinder)

Inadequate Spacers

Other devices place distance between the patient's mouth and the MDI but they are not true spacers as the volume is too small or they do not have a valved chamber. They do not remove the need for precise timing in the actuation of the MDI, and only allow a little more time for inhalation. They are not recommended as they only give an illusion of better inhalation. Examples include the following:

- MicroSpacer
- Mist-Assist
- Azmacort has an included spacer
- Dixie Cup with a hole (or similar improvisation). Since this is open at both ends, there is significant loss of medication to the air

Tips for Using Spacers

- A spacer with mask can be useful for infants and young children, but effective use requires parental education. Despite controversy in the literature, it is probably not a substitute for a nebulizer unit in younger patients or patients in acute distress. It is not uncommon for patients to do well in the office, but their technique slips when they are at home or having acute problems.
- Older children (over 8–10 years) can usually learn open-mouth technique, especially with HFA units.
- For the sake of consistency, spacers should always be used for inhaled steroids as this minimizes complications such as oral candidiasis and dysphonia. Even with use of a spacer with inhaled steroids, patients should be instructed to rinse their mouth after inhalation, or to use the medication prior to brushing their teeth.

Dry Powder Devices

Structure

The underlying principle of these devices is constant even though the design varies, but there is little uniformity in the mechanism from one device to another. The technique remains consistent.

Method

Essentially, the medication is stored in a powdered form, and a propellant is not used. The device is primed by cocking a lever, rotating a disk or puncturing a blister package or a capsule. The dose then becomes available in a delivery chamber. The patient inhales directly from this chamber. Timing is not a critical issue, as with MDIs, as the medication is only delivered when the patient inhales. The patient does not have to allow for the high nozzle speed that is found in MDIs. With all of these devices, the patient inhales through the mouthpiece from full exhalation to full inhalation with a 10-second breath hold at the end.

Examples

Diskus. This is an easy to use delivery device. As the name implies, this device is disc shaped. The medication is stored on a roll in blisters at regular intervals. Opening the unit and priming by drawing a lever back punctures one of the blisters and decreases the number on a counter by one. The medication drops into the delivery chamber, and is inhaled from there. The device must be held horizontally. The patient must be instructed not to blow into the device.

Type of medications that use this device:

Serevent (salmeterol)

- One puff of powder (50 µg) equals two inhalations of the MDI form of the drug.
- Since the powder has lactose filler, the patient is aware of receiving the dose.
- The unit holds 50 doses.

Advair (salmeterol and fluticasone). Advair is a combination drug that contains fluticasone (Flovent) and salmeterol. There are data that indicate that administering the two drugs simultaneously provides a therapeutic advantage. This is a useful combination for patients with asthma who continue to have symptoms, such as nocturnal cough or exercise symptoms.

There are three strengths: fluticasone/salmeterol = 100/50, 250/50, 500/50 µg.

Pulmicort turbuhaler. This device is specific for budesonide, a long acting and potent corticosteroid.

The Turbuhaler is a tube shaped device with internal vanes that direct the medication into a tight spiral, theoretically allowing for deeper penetration into the lungs. The medication is kept in a holding chamber. When a disk at the bottom is rotated, a measured amount of the medication drops into one of five delivery chambers. The patient needs to generate a stronger inhalation force than with the Diskus. Inspiratory effort must be about 30–40 L/min. Patient barely perceives the dose, which can be a problem. The canister contains 200 doses. Unlike the Diskus, this device does not have a counter, but relies on a sliding gauge that turns red when there are 10 doses left.

A trainer whistle is available. This is similar to the actual device. Patients should be reminded that the actual device does not make a noise.

Flovent rotadisk. A disk containing four blister package doses of fluticasone fits into a powder delivery device. This is a cumbersome device that is based on old technology. The delivery is adequate, but there may be significant loss of medication. Powder tends to adhere to the inside of the device. The disk is placed into the Dischaler by opening a slide. The device is closed, and the blister is punctured by lifting a lever. The same inhalation technique is used as for other dry powder inhalers.

The blister packages contain four doses of fluticasone. There are three strengths (50, 100, and 250 µg per puff).

Foradil aerolizer. This is a device that is specific for formoterol, a long-acting beta agonist. It is based on old technology. The medication is kept in separate capsules, which are placed in a chamber within a plastic holder with a mouthpiece. The capsule is punctured using two buttons on the side of the inhaler. The patient inhales with a moderate force to maximal inhalation and holds his/her breath for 10 seconds. If there is doubt about the completeness of inhalation, the device can be opened to check if the medication is completely inhaled. If not, a second inhalation is taken after closing the device. Keeping the medication and device separately raises the potential for losing one or both. Too many steps are needed for complete inhalation of the medication, making it difficult for children or elderly patients.

Education regarding proper spacer use in the office

- Have the spacer device in the office to show a patient and family.
- Use some careful in-office instructions as with education regarding MDI without spacer (see above).
- Ideally, the time between actuation of the canister and inhalation should be short. This is less critical with true valved spacers.
- The canister needs to be well shaken.
- The patient should place the spacer in his/her mouth ready to inhale and then depress the canister.
- The patient should take a steady breath to maximal inhalation and hold for 10 seconds. Have the patient exhale, and take a second breath from the spacer.
- The patient should then take a second dose in the same manner. Emphasize to the patient not to use more than one spray into the spacer at a time.
- Wash the spacer in weak dishwasher soap solution and dry well to keep clean approximately every week. The bag of the InspirEase should never be washed, but replaced on a monthly basis. The EZ Spacer bag is washable and should last for 1 year. The patient should probably have two spacers to use one while the other is drying.
- Check technique every time the patient comes to the office.

Nebulizer Therapy

A nebulizer is a device that generates a mist from a solution of the medication that a patient inhales from a mouthpiece or face mask. Nebulizers are a very inefficient form of medication delivery, and the starting dose of medication is usually higher than is delivered by MDIs at the mouthpiece. The inefficiency is offset by ease of use. The loss of medication is compensated by a longer delivery time than other devices and a higher starting dose.

Medication delivery is by mouthpiece or mask. Parents should be discouraged from using so called "blow by" method. This involves holding the end of the delivery tube near the child's face. The delivery of medication by this method is extremely poor. The mouthpiece is the best delivery choice for older patients, and a mask for infants and young children. A nebulizer is also useful for elderly or disabled patients who cannot manage another form of delivery, such as MDI.

Method

General method. There are three ways to have a patient inhale nebulizer mist:

- Mouthpieces
- Mask
- "Blow by" (sometimes used for young children). This is a very ineffective method and should be actively discouraged

Formulations

- Medications available for nebulizer are listed in Table 14-1.
- Most medication comes prediluted in volumes of 2.0–3.0 cc, except for albuterol in bulk packaging which needs to be diluted in normal or half-normal saline to a volume of 3 cc. Bronchosaline (a bulk saline dispenser) is commercially available OTC and is less expensive than vials of normal saline. Undiluted albuterol concentrate can be used with an ultrasonic nebulizer only.
- Diluting the medication changes the effective concentration that reaches the airway. The actual dose that is received is a function of minute ventilation. The longer the nebulization lasts, the more medication the patients will receive.
- Try to have the patient take deep breaths. Proper coaching is essential.
- Since the therapy takes a long time, the parents can try to make the nebulization experience positive every time by reading a book to the child or watching TV together.

TABLE 14-1

LIST OF THE MOST FREQUENTLY USED MEDICATIONS FOR ADMINISTRATION USING A NEBULIZER

Generic Name	Action	Concentration
Albuterol	Beta$_2$ agonist	0.083% premixed
		0.5% (0.5 mL/3 mL saline)
Levalbuterol	Beta$_2$ agonist—isomer	0.31 mg/3 mL
		0.63 mg/3 mL
		1.25 mg/3 mL
Budesonide	Steroid	0.25 mg/2 mL
		0.5 mg/2 mL
Ipratropium	Anticholinergic	0.5 mg/2.5 mL
Glycopyrrolate	Anticholinergic	0.2 mg/mL

Types of Nebulizer

There are two types of nebulizer: pressure driven (jet or venturi) or ultrasonic.

Jet. Jet nebulizers utilize the Venturi principle of flow by forcing the liquid through a small opening thereby breaking it into a fine mist. Ideally, the resultant particles size should range around 5 μm . There are differences among nebulizer designs. Some medications are more dependent on the design than are others. One should rely on the manufacturers' information. In general, though, there is considerable waste of medication in a nebulizer, and the effect of different designs is often immaterial.

Ultrasonic. Because ultrasonic nebulizers break up the liquids by sound energy, and tend to produce a more uniform particle size. Medications that are in the form of a suspension (e.g., Pulmicort Respules) cannot be delivered by an ultrasonic device. Realistically, however, there is probably no difference in delivery between ultrasonic and jet systems. Most ultrasonic devices do not have face-masks, so they are not suitable for young children. This system uses a smaller volume of medication than the jet nebulizer does.

Advantages

- Nebulized therapy is ideal for use by young children who cannot use MDIs. It is also the method of choice in an acute situation where a patient cannot use an MDI effectively.
- Nebulizers eliminate the need for precise technique.
- This method delivers a high dose of medication slowly, allowing more time for absorption and lung deposition. Some of the medication may be absorbed sublingually, producing high blood levels because of avoiding a first pass through the liver.
- One should have a low "threshold" to get a family of a child with asthma a nebulizer for home use. It is the ideal delivery system for a child having an acute asthmatic episode, and early therapy is the key to keeping asthmatics out of the emergency department and hospital. Saving on only one emergency department visit easily covers the cost of the machine ($150.00).

Disadvantages

- This method is slow, taxing the patience of small children. A treatment can last 10–15 minutes, depending on the machine. Ultrasonic nebulizers are faster.
- While several studies indicate that there may not be advantages compared to well-used MDI, a nebulizer is probably still the most efficient method in small children, elderly or arthritic patients, patients who are mentally retarded,

and patients in acute respiratory distress. Both methods will deliver about 10% of the dose below the glottis.

Maintaining Nebulizer/Compressor

- Wash nebulizer bowl with diluted soap and water every few days if used regularly.
- Alternate two nebulizer bowls.
- Change compressor filter every few months if used often.

All pediatric offices should have at least one nebulizer for use in the office for children with acute asthma. If possible, there should also be a "loaner" machine available to patients for short-term use at home.

SPECIFIC MEDICATIONS

Sympathomimetics

Several new products have appeared on the market. The latest have half-lives that range from 4 to 12 hours and have good $\beta2$ specificity.

Common Side Effects

The members of this group of medications resemble each other in their range of side effects. They differ in degree, with older drugs, like isoproterenol, having more marked effects and newer derivatives, like levalbuterol, having fewer. Common side effects are shown in Table 14-2.

TABLE 14-2

COMMON SIDE EFFECTS OF THE BETA AGONISTS ARE LISTED

Tremor
Nausea
Tachycardia
Palpitations
Nervousness and agitation
Increased blood pressure
Dizziness
Heartburn

Beta Agonist Controversy

The NAEPP currently recommends that $\beta2$ agonists should only be used as needed for acute asthma episodes. There are studies (Spitzer et al.) that indicate that patients who use albuterol on a regular basis actually do not do as well as those who use the medication only to relieve acute symptoms. Several studies have indicated that patients who used more than two canisters of a β agonist per month were at greater risk of morbidity and mortality. There is a controversy about concluding from these studies that this outcome was the result of excessive use of the beta agonist. These data are more likely to indicate that the patients needed steroids or other anti-inflammatory drugs as a controller medication. Put differently, the same high risk outcome can occur in patients who are not on controller medications.

Mullen et al. supported this conclusion in an extensive review of case controlled studies. Their analysis indicated that there was no association between the frequency of β agonist use and higher morbidity or mortality.

Types of Beta Agonists

There are several preparations available with similar activities. These are shown on Table 14-3. Older preparations, such as isoproterenol, have a short duration of action, but are potent agonists.

Oral

Oral beta agonists are formulated to deliver 2 mg in 5 mL or as 2 or 4 mg tablets.

The oral route is very inefficient as a means of delivering beta agonists. Side effects are common and troublesome, especially in children. This is not a recommended route of administration. There are few indications to use this approach.

Nebulized

This form of administration is useful in younger children, the elderly, and patients who are having acute distress.

Xopenex (levalbuterol) is an isomeric form of albuterol. It is R(-)albuterol, and is physically the right hand (R) form and optically is levorotatory (-).

TABLE 14-3

THE TYPES OF BETA AGONIST BRONCHODILATORS ARE SHOWN, WITH THE PREPARATIONS AND DURATION OF ACTION

Generic Name	Trade Name	Preparations	Duration	Unusual Features
Albuterol	Ventolin Proventil	Oral 2 mg/5 mL 2, 4 mg tabs MDI 90 μg/spray Proventil HFA 108 μg/spray Nebulizer 2.5 mg/3 mL	4 hours	
Terbutaline	Brethine	Oral 2.5, 5 mg tabs Parenteral 1 mg/mL	4 hours	Used IV in severe asthma
Levalbuterol	Xopenex	Nebulizer 0.31 mg/3 mL 0.63 mg/3 mL 1.25 mg/3 mL	4–8 hours	Pure isomer of albuterol
Pirbuterol	Maxair Autohaler	MDI 200 μg/spray	4 hours	Breath actuated
Isoproterenol	Isuprel	IV	1–2 hours	IV in severe asthma β1 activity
Epinephrine		Parenteral 1:1000 (1 mg/ mL)	10–15 minutes	Subcutaneous or IM in severe asthma
Salmeterol	Serevent	Diskus (DPI) 50 μg/inhalation	12 hours	Never use for rescue Long acting airway control
Formoterol	Foradil	Aerolizer 12 μg/inhalation	12 hours	Never use for rescue Long acting airway control

Note: Some have unusual features that are specifically mentioned in this table.

The S-albuterol isomer may have bronchoconstrictive properties and be deleterious to airway function. Levalbuterol produces as much bronchodilation as racemic albuterol at doses as low as 0.31 mg/3 mL versus 2.5 mg/3 mL of racemic albuterol. Fewer side effects, such as tachycardia, are reported with levalbuterol.

Metered Dose Inhaler

Currently, albuterol (Ventolin, Proventil) and pirbuterol (Maxair Autohaler) are available as a metered dose inhaler. The propellant, chlorofluorocarbon has been banned, and a substitute will replace it. Proventil HFA contains an alternative propellant, tetrafluoroethane, and other devices will follow.

Albuterol

Max heart rate 1.5x resting following dose

> *Oral.* 0.1 mg/kg; max 12 mg/day
> *Inhaled.*
>> *Nebulized:* 2.5 mg/3 mL. Since inhaled medications are self-titrated by minute ventilation, there is no reason to dose based on the patient's weight
>> *MDI:* Two sprays every 4–8 hours (with a spacer in children or patients who cannot master MDI technique)

Salmeterol

- Salmeterol is a beta agonist with duration of action of 12 hours. Salmeterol is modified from the basic albuterol molecule with the addition of a long side chain that decreases catabolism. This chain also distorts the molecule, reducing binding efficiency to the beta receptor. The partial binding makes salmeterol an incomplete agonist, delaying the onset of action. This drug is very useful in patients with nocturnal and exercise induced symptoms because of the prolonged action.
- Salmeterol should never be used for rescue therapy.

Formoterol. This is a long acting agonist that is effective for at least 12 hours. Unlike salmeterol, formoterol is a complete agonist with a rapid onset of action. It is useful for nocturnal symptoms and exercise induced asthma. It is currently only available in a capsule dry powder form. The device that is used (see Aerolizer above) is complicated to operate and only moderately efficient. Formoterol is available in Canada and Europe in combination with budesonide, but this form is not approved in the United States as of this writing. A summary of beta agonists is given in Table 14-3.

Steroids

General

Glucocorticoids are the mainstay of control of chronic inflammatory disorders such as asthma and allergic rhinitis. They have a wide range of effects on cells and mediators of inflammation. If steroids need to be used for a longer period to control symptoms, the patient should be weaned to an alternate day dose schedule. Topical preparations have the best balance of efficacy and side effects. Topical forms of steroids are available for skin, for inhalation and as nasal preparations. Topical use allows for the use of a much lower concentration than is needed orally.

Effects of Glucocorticoids

Cells. Steroids have a major effect in increasing the availability of beta receptors on smooth muscle and other cells, thus enhancing the action of beta agonist medications.

Lymphocytes are trapped in lymphatics, resulting in decreased circulatory numbers. Steroids block interactions between lymphocytes and macrophages (for example, the response to tuberculin in the PPD reaction).

Polymorphonuclear cells increase in number by two-thirds in peripheral blood, because of demargination within blood vessels. Normally, two-thirds of polymorphonuclear cells are attached to blood vessel walls (marginated) preparatory to moving into the perivascular space. There is reduced fluidity of the cell membrane, and decreased ability of the polymorphonuclear cells to form pseudopods and migrate from blood. The loss of membrane fluidity also decreases the ability of the neutrophils to engulf organisms in pinocytic vacuoles, potentially reducing their immune function.

Eosinophil numbers decrease markedly in peripheral blood.

Macrophage mediator release is inhibited.

Platelet membranes are stabilized, decreasing normal destruction in the spleen.

Steroids have minimal effects on mast cells in vivo, and do not significantly block the release of histamine or leukotrienes in clinical trials. In vitro, there is inhibition of the release of arachidonic acid metabolites and platelet activating factor.

At inflammatory sites. There is a reduction of the *influx* of inflammatory cells, mainly because of the reduction of chemokines that attract several classes of inflammatory cells.

Steroids inhibit *proinflammatory cytokines* (interleukin-1 [IL1], IL4, IL13, IL16).

Blood vessels. There is a decrease in transudation of fluid across capillaries and resultant edema formation.

Miscellaneous effects. Steroids increase the production of surfactants from the lungs and decrease the mucus content, improving lung function.

Steroid Formulations

General. Duration of action

> *Onset:* In general, it takes 4–6 hours for the effects of a steroid dose to become apparent. The duration of action of a single dose is around 6 hours
>
> Dosing should be set to coincide with the normal diurnal peaks of cortisol, at 8 AM and at 3 PM. The larger peak is at 8 AM, and this is the optimal time to give a single daily dose

Oral

Prednisone. Prednisone is a prodrug that is catabolized in the liver to prednisolone and an inert component. It may be less effective if the patient has a problem with hepatic function.

Dose

> For asthma and other allergic disorders, dosing is usually by weight
>
> *Loading dose:* 2 mg/kg to maximum 60–80 mg/day
>
> *Continue:* 1 mg/kg to maximum 60–80 mg/day
>
> These limits are recommended in the NAEPP. Higher doses have been shown to increase the risk of side effects without adding significantly to the patient's response
>
> A common dose schedule is for 5 days, after which the drug can be discontinued without tapering. While adrenal suppression can be seen after a short course of steroids, they usually recover within a few weeks
>
> *Frequency:* There does not seem to be much difference between daily or twice daily dosing

Duration of therapy

> Usually 3–7 days, then stop (no taper)
>
> 7+ days; rapid taper by 5–10 mg/day
>
> Chronic steroids; gradual taper to every other day then discontinue as condition allows
>
> *Formulations:*
>
> > *Tablets:* 1, 2.5, 5, 10, 20, 50 mg
> >
> > *Suspension:* 5/5, 15/5, 25 mg/5mL

Prednisolone. The active formulation of prednisone is available in liquid form under several brand names (Prelone, Orapred, Pediapred and generic). It is better tasting than prednisone.

Methylprednisolone (Medrol). Medrol is similar to prednisone, with a ratio Medrol:Prednisone as 4:5.

Medrol has an advantage in having very little mineralocorticoid activity. As a result, there are fewer side effects, such as myalgia, headache, and mood swings. In liquid preparations, it is better tasting than prednisone, and is tolerated by children. It is generally much more costly than Prednisone.

> *Formulations:*
>
> > *Tablets:* 2, 4, 8, 16, 24, 32 mg
> >
> > *Parenteral:* For IV use. Generally given in acute asthma, 1–2 mg/kg/day divided q6–q8 hours

Alternate day use of steroids. If steroids are required for a longer period to control severe symptoms of asthma or urticaria and angioedema, the side effects can be reduced considerably by shifting to an alternate day dose schedule. Start at high dose to gain control of the patient's symptoms and then decrease dose slowly as tolerated. Begin the taper once the symptoms are under control, with a minimum of 5 days of oral steroid.

There are many methods of converting the patient to an alternate day regimen. The exact method used probably matters less than maintaining control and proceeding slowly. From a pathophysiologic perspective, one is allowing the inflammation to escape control by the steroid, and giving the next dose before the inflammation becomes clinically relevant. As a result, patients can break through the control of alternate day dosing quite easily and should be closely monitored.

TABLE 14-4

TAPERING SCHEDULES FOR PREDNISONE

A

Day	1	2	3	4	5	6	7	8	9	10	
Dose mg	60	55	50	45	40	35	30	25	20	15	
Day	11	12	13	14	15	16	17	18	19	20	
Dose mg	20	10	20	5	20	0	20	0	20	0	

B

Day	1	2	3	4	5	6	7	8	9	10	
Dose mg	60	55	50	45	40	35	30	25	20	25	
Day	11	12	13	14	15	16	17	18	19	20	
Dose mg	15	30	10	35	5	40	0	40	0	40	

C

Day	21	22	23	24	25	26	27	28	29	30	31
Dose mg	40	0	35	0	35	0	35	0	30	0	30
Day	32	33	34	35	36	37	38	39	40	41	42
Dose mg	0	30	0	25	0	25	0	25	0	20	0

Note: A: A suggested taper for moderate disease symptoms in patients who have frequent acute episodes or have had a more severe acute episode that requires prolonged therapy. B: A suggested taper for patients with more severe disease. C: A tapering schedule to an every other day dose in patients who have refractory disease such as chronic urticaria or severe asthma. This type of taper provides steroid control while minimizing side effects. This table is only intended as a guide. Actual dose depends on severity and must be tailored to each patient based on age, weight, and severity of disease.

One dosing schedule is to decrease by 5 mg daily until the patient is at 20 mg daily. The dose can be held at 20 mg one day and decreased on the alternate day until the patient is at 20 mg every other day. The alternate day dose can then be tapered as tolerated.

The following tables are intended as a guide. Dosing should be tapered according to an individual patient's needs. Three dosing guides are given in Table 14-4.

Approximate alternate daily doses for refractory patients could be:

1 year	10 mg qod
1–4 years	20 mg qod
5–12 years	30 mg qod
>12 years	40 mg qod

Side effects of oral steroids. The severity of untoward effects of oral steroid therapy is proportional to the duration of therapy.

The most frequent are noted; this is not an exhaustive list. Increased appetite, nausea, and weight gain are the most common. Patients may develop a cushingoid appearance with centripetal obesity, facial swelling, and a buffalo hump. Hirsutism occurs commonly. Headache, mood swings, and lethargy are often reported. Fluid and electrolyte disturbances may occur particularly with sodium retention and there is a risk of hypokalemia.

Side effects of steroids are listed in Table 14-5.

Inhaled steroids. The availability of potent, safe, inhaled steroids that have long half-lives has had a significant effect on control of asthma. The inhaled steroids can be considered as older, short acting and lower potency or newer, long acting, and high potency. These medications are not comparable on a milligram for milligram basis. The NAEPP presents doses for these steroids as low, medium and high dose ranges, rather than making a direct comparison. These and related tables can be found at http://www.nhlbi.nih.gov/health/prof/lung/index.htm #asthma

SIDE EFFECT OF ORAL STEROID THERAPY

Musculoskeletal:
Growth suppression in children
    Correlates with dose and duration of therapy
Myalgia
Aseptic necrosis of femoral and humeral heads
Muscle weakness
Loss of muscle mass
Myopathy
Osteoporosis
Pathologic fractures
Vertebral compression fractures

Gastrointestinal
Peptic ulcer (possible hemorrhage and perforation)
Pancreatitis
Ulcerative esophagitis

Dermatologic
Facial erythema
Impaired wound healing
Suppress t cell-macrophage reactions to skin tests
Striae
Petechiae and ecchymoses
Thin fragile skin
Edema

Neurological
Headache
Pseudotumor cerebri usually when discontinuing
treatment
Convulsions
Psychic disorders
Vertigo
Glaucoma
Cataracts (posterior lenticular cataracts are typical
of steroids)

Endocrine
Adrenocortical suppression
Risk of shock in response to stress
Decreased carbohydrate tolerance
Revealing latent diabetes
Menstrual irregularities

Note: Most side effects relate to prolonged use. Over the short term, untoward effects usually reverse.

For example, fluticasone low dose = 88–264 μg, medium dose = 264–660 μg, high dose = >660 μg and budesonide low dose = 200–400 μg, medium dose = 400–600 μg, high dose = >600 μg. By contrast, the dose ranges for a lower potency steroid, flunisolide, low dose = 500–1000 μg, medium dose = 1000–2000 μg, high dose = >2000 μg. In addition, lower potency steroids usually require every 8-hour dosing, while higher potency drugs can be given once to twice daily. Broad groupings according to potency are given in Table 14-6.

Lower potency

Beclomethasone diproprionate: This compound is rapidly broken down to the active monoproprionate form at the mucosal surface. A newer form of this agent is QVAR, which is beclomethasone in an MDI format with HFA propellant, rather than CFC.

Dose: 42, 84 μg per actuation
Preparations: Ventolin, Beclovent, generic
Nasal formulations (Beconase, Vancenase)

Triamcinolone:
Preparation: Azmacort
Dose: 100 μg/actuation
Azmacort has a fold up "spacer" that allows more time for inhalation. This drug is less useful than newer agents, such as budesonide. It requires tid dosing
Nasal formulations (Nasacort AQ)

High potency

Fluticasone proprionate: Fluticasone is a potent, long-acting steroid molecule that is highly lipophilic and binds firmly to the steroid receptor. It provides 12–24 hours of anti-inflammatory action.

Dose:
    MDI: 44, 110, 220 mg per actuation
    Advair Diskus: fluticasone/salmeterol 100/50, 250/50, 500/50 mg
    Rotadisk: 50, 100, 250 μg
Delivery: MDI, DPI (Rotadisk, Diskus)
Preparations: Flovent, Advair (Flovent + salmeterol)
Nasal formulation (Flonase)

TABLE 14-6

BROAD GROUPING OF INHALED CORTICOSTEROIDS BY WHETHER THEY ARE OF LOW POTENCY AND SHORT DURATION OR OF HIGHER POTENCY AND LONGER DURATION

Lower potency, short duration	*Higher potency, long duration*
Beclomethasone (Beclovent)	Fluticasone (Flovent)
Flunisolide (AeroBid)	Budesonide (Pulmicort)
Triamcinolone (Azmacort)	Mometasone (Azmanex—not yet released)

Note: Potency is measured by inhibition of vascular permeability and does not encompass the full range of steroid anti-inflammatory effects.

Budesonide. Budesonide has an unusual metabolic pathway. It exists in a balance of water and fat soluble forms. It is stored in the water soluble form, and as the lipid soluble molecule is consumed by the steroid receptor, the balance shifts in favor of the lipid soluble form.

It binds strongly to the steroid receptor, and provides 12–24 hours of anti-inflammatory effect.

Dose:
    Pulmicort Turbuhaler: 200 μg/inhalation
    Pulmicort Respules: 250, 500 μg per vial
Delivery:
    DPI—Turbuhaler
    Nebulizer—Respules
In moderate to severe asthmatics, the approach should be to start at a high dose and decrease slowly as tolerated. In mild asthmatics, one can start with a low dose (44 μg 200 μg budesonide daily) and increase if needed
Nasal formulation (Rhinocort aqua)

Side effects of inhaled steroids

In general, these are safe drugs.

Local complications: Local complications are the most common. Dysphonia and oral thrush can be frequent, but are prevented by rinsing the mouth after inhaling the medication. Advising the patient to use the medication after brushing their teeth also serves as a reminder to take it.

Inhaled steroids should always be taken with a spacer (Aerochamber or InspirEase) when an MDI is used. It is not needed for DPIs.

Systemic complications: As with any chronic steroid, there may be *adrenal suppression*. This is a dose dependent complication, and the frequency rises rapidly as the dose is increased. The clinical significance is not clear, and usually there is recovery when the dose is reduced or the drug is discontinued. Patients exhibit varied sensitivity to steroids, especially fluticasone. They may develop *increased appetite, weight gain, and mood swings*. In children, growth velocity should be monitored, and the dose reduced or the patient changed to a less potent steroid if there is a *reduction in growth rate*. Long-term studies indicate that children on chronic budesonide attain predicted height.

Most of the studies that have shown decreased growth velocity in children and bone demineralization in adults have been on high doses of potent steroids (3–4 mg/day), but patients may develop side effects as an idiosyncratic sensitivity. Any patient on chronic inhaled steroids should have a periodic slit lamp examination to monitor for *cataracts*.

Nasal preparations: Nasal use of steroids carries a low risk of systemic complications. Local effects include nasal drying and epistaxis.

Dermatologic preparations. Topical steroids are categorized by potency based on the induction of vasoconstriction. There are seven levels of potency, with I most potent and VII least. Since preparations in each category have similar profiles, choice within a category is a matter of preference and patient

TABLE 14-7

EXAMPLES ARE GIVEN OF TOPICAL STEROIDS IN EACH OF SEVEN POTENCY GROUPS, WITH I AS MOST POTENT AND VII AS LEAST

Group	Brand Name	Percent	Generic Name	Tube Size (gm; Unless Noted)
I	Ultravate cream, ointment	0.05	Halobetasol propionate	15, 50
	Diprolene lotion, ointment, gel	0.05	Augmented betamethasone dipropionate	30, 60 mL
II	Alphatrex ointment	0.05	Betamethasone dipropionate	15, 45
III	Aristocort cream, ointment	0.5	Triamcinolone acetonide	15, 240
	Elocon ointment	0.1	Mometasone furoate	15, 45
IV	Kenalog ointment	0.1	Triamcinolone acetonide	15, 60, 80, 240, 2520
	Synalar ointment	0.025	Fluocinolone acetonide	15, 30, 60, 120, 425
V	Aristocort cream	0.1	Triamcinolone acetonide	15, 60, 240, 2520
	Cutivate cream	0.05	Fluticasone propionate	15, 30, 60
VI	Aristocort cream	0.025	Triamcinolone acetonide	15, 60, 240, 2520
	Kenalog cream, lotion	0.025	Triamcinolone acetonide	15, 60, 80, 240, 2520
VII	Celestone cream	0.2	Betamethasone valerate	15
	Synacort cream	1.0	Hydrocortisone	15, 30, 60
		2.5		30

tolerance. The most common examples in each category are presented in Table 14-7.

There are several vehicles for the steroids, the most usual being cream, ointment, lotion, and gel.

Creams. The cream base is an emulsification of oils and water with a preservative. Creams may be irritating or cause reactions to components. They are best used on wet areas, because they have a tendency to cause dryness. They are often used in the groin and intertriginous areas. They have the advantage of not staining clothing and being cosmetically acceptable. The key characteristics are the following:

- White in color and somewhat greasy texture
- Contain components that may cause irritation, stinging, and allergy

- High versatility (i.e., may be used in nearly any area), therefore creams are the base most often prescribed
- Cosmetically most acceptable, particularly emollient bases (e.g., Lidex-E, Topicort, and Cyclocort)
- Possible drying effect with continued use, therefore best for acute exudative inflammation
- Most useful for intertriginous areas (e.g., groin, rectal area, and axilla)

Ointments. The ointment base contains a limited number of organic compounds consisting primarily of greases such as petroleum jelly, with little or no water. Many ointments are preservative-free. Ointments have the following characteristics:

- Translucent (look like petroleum jelly)
- Greasy feeling persists on skin surface
- More lubrication, thus desirable for drier lesions
- Greater penetration of medicine than creams and therefore enhanced potency (see inside front cover; Synalar Cream in group V and Synalar Ointment in group IV)
- Too occlusive for acute (exudative) eczematous inflammation or intertriginous areas, such as the groin

Gels. Gels are greaseless mixtures of propylene glycol and water; some also contain alcohol. Gels have the following characteristics:

- A clear base, sometimes with a jellylike consistency
- Useful for acute exudative inflammation, such as poison ivy, and in scalp areas where other vehicles mat the hair

Solutions and lotions. Solutions may contain water and alcohol as well as other chemicals. Solutions have the following characteristics:

- Clear or milky appearance
- Most useful for scalp because they penetrate easily through hair, leaving no residue
- May result in stinging and drying when applied to intertriginous areas, such as the groin

Aerosols. Aerosols are composed of steroids suspended in a base and delivered under pressure. Aerosols have the following characteristics:

- Useful for applying medication to the scalp (long probe attached to the can may be inserted through the hair to deliver medication more easily to the scalp)
- Useful for moist lesions such as poison ivy
- Convenient for patients who lack mobility and have difficulty reaching their lower legs

Potency. There are seven levels of cutaneous potency of steroids, with I as most potent and VII as least. In this instance, potency is measured as the inhibition of vascular permeability. Only selected common examples in each category are given in Table14-7.

Theophylline

The methylxanthines, particularly dimethylxanthine (theophylline) have been successfully used in asthma. The overall benefit, however, is probably weak, and there is a high side-effect profile. Side effects include gastrointestinal upset, sleeplessness, headache, shortened attention span in children, and tachycardia.

Theophylline has fallen into disuse, primarily because of the high side-effect profile. The potential for low dose theophylline to function as a steroid sparing drug is being reexamined. Theophylline may act as a weak anti-inflammatory agent, and has some bronchodilator effect.

Dose

Administer q 12 hours as an acceptable slow-release product.

Most children under 8 years require q 8 hour dosing.

Titrate to final dose over 1-week period (use ideal body weight)

<1 year	blood level is unpredictable-caution
1–9 years	22 mg/kg/day
9–12 years	20 mg/kg/day
12–16 years	18 mg/kg/day
>16 years	13 mg/kg/day
Maximum dose	900 mg/day
Loading dose maximum	400 mg/day

Check serum concentration and adjust dose to keep at 10–20 μg/mL. A lower level that is consistent with clinical control is acceptable. The use of theophylline in an acute asthma episode has not proved to be better in decreasing morbidity or in preventing or decreasing the length of a hospital admission than placebo.

Cromolyn Sodium (Intal)

Cromolyn inhibits mast cell disintegration in response to allergen exposure. It stabilizes mast cell and other inflammatory cell membranes.

This drug has limited use by inhalation, and has been supplanted by the more effective leukotriene modifiers. While safe, the inhaled form (nebulized or MDI) is only moderately effective in preventing bronchospasm. It may require 4–6 weeks to become effective.

Formulations

Nebulizer solution

20 mg tid-qid. Generic only available
MDI—Two puffs via metered dose inhaler (with spacer) tid-qid

Oral. 100 mg capsules or 100 mg/5 mL solution used in severe allergic gastritis or esophagitis

Opthalmic. 4% solution. This is particularly effective in vernal conjunctivitis

Side Effects

Diarrhea, nausea, abdominal pain, constipation, dyspepsia, flatulence, glossitis, stomatitis, vomiting.

Nedocromil Sodium (Tilade)

Nedocromil is an inflammatory cell stabilizing drug. It affects mast cells, basophils, eosinophils, and neutrophils.

It has a longer duration of action than cromolyn, and may have a greater effectiveness.

Formulations

MDI. Two puffs qid. May be reduced to bid once symptoms are controlled. Each actuation delivers 2.0 mg of nedocromil.

Ophthalmic preparation. (Alocril) 2% solution. This preparation is useful in allergic and vernal conjunctivitis.

Anticholinergic Agents

Currently the use of inhaled anticholinergic agents is only approved for chronic obstructive lung disease in adults. Nevertheless, there are data to indicate that anticholinergic agents are useful in relieving acute bronchospasm in asthma, especially in refractory acute situations. Common types of anticholinergics are shown in Table 14-8.

TABLE 14-8

DOSING OF THE ANTICHOLINERGIC AGENTS

Medication	Inhaled dose
Atropine	250–500 μg q6 h
Glycopyrrolate	0.05 mg/kg q6 h
Ipratropium bromide	0.01–0.05 mg/kg q6h

Ipratropium

Nebulized. Ipratropium in a nebulized format is frequently used in the acute situation. It is supplied as 500 mg/2.5 mL. The usual dose is one vial every 6–8 hours by inhalation. Once the patient improves, the frequency is usually reduced. There is little benefit outside of the acute situation, and anticholinergic medications do not have any prophylactic benefit in asthma. Anticholinergic preparations are particularly useful in cough that has an asthmatic or allergic cause.

Nasal. Ipratropium is useful in nasal congestion in allergic rhinitis. It is supplied in an aqueous spray as 0.03 and 0.06%, and is used bid to tid.

Glycopyrrolate

Glycopyrrolate (Robinul) is also used for the acute episode. The nebulized format that is available is also a parenteral solution, which is nebulized. The medication is available in an oral preparation as 1 and 2 mg strengths. The oral form is useful to control secretions and to help with cough.

Anti-IgE

A newly released product, omalizumab (Xolair) is a recombinant humanized IgG monoclonal antibody that selectively binds to human immunoglobulin E (IgE). It is administered by the subcutaneous route once to twice per month. There is no finite limit to the duration of therapy.

Mechanism of Action

Omalizumab inhibits the binding of IgE to the high-affinity IgE receptor (FcεRI) on the surface of mast cells and basophils, which limits the release of inflammatory mediators.

In clinical studies, serum free IgE levels were reduced >96% within 1 hour following the first dose and maintained between doses. Mean serum free IgE decrease was greater than 96% using recommended doses. There is an initial rise in serum IgE levels. Total IgE levels do not return to pretreatment levels for up to 1 year after discontinuation of omalizumab. Studies in moderate to severe asthmatics indicate reduction of acute episodes of asthma with use of Xolair, but no change in hospitalization rates. Xolair may have potential for use in patients with severe food allergy.

Indication

Omalizumab is indicated for adults and adolescents (12 years of age and above) with moderate to severe persistent asthma who have a positive skin test or in vitro reactivity to a perennial aeroallergen and whose symptoms are inadequately controlled with inhaled corticosteroids.

Methotrexate

There is some indication that the use of antimetabolite drugs can lead to reducing the dose of steroid and improved outcome in severe patients. These drugs should be reserved for severe, refractory patients only and should be administered under the supervision of a specialist.

BLOCKERS OF MEDIATORS

Antihistamines

This group of medications may be the most used, considering OTC and prescription drugs. They can be classified as sedating and nonsedating. The sedating antihistamines belong to an older generation, while newer compounds cause much less sedation.

Actions

Antihistamines have a wide range of actions. The most prominent is in blocking histamine H1 receptors. They also decrease release of other chemical mediators of inflammation including PGD2, LTC4, kinins, and tryptase from mast cells and basophils. There is decreased chemotaxis and activation of eosinophils, neutrophils, and basophils. Reduced adhesion protein expression has also been noted. Anti-inflammatory effects are seen at higher than normal doses of the antihistamine. Many antihistamines also have anticholinergic and antiserotonin properties.

Blockers of H2 receptors are useful in chronic urticaria because of the presence of H2 receptors in blood vessels. Examples are cimetidine (Tagamet) and ranitidine (Zantac). Both are dosed at 150 mg bid or 4–5 mg/kg/day in divided doses.

Sedating Antihistamines

Common examples

Diphenhydramine (Benadryl) tablets 25, 50 mg, 12.5 mg/5 mL liquid
Hydroxyzine (Atarax, Vistaril) tablets 25, 50 mg, 10 mg/5 mL
Cyproheptadine (Periactin) tablets 4 mg, 2 mg/5 mL
Chlorpheniramine or Brompheniramine (numerous OTC preparations) 4, 8, 12 mg

The sedating antihistamines are generally similar in duration of action from 4 to 6 hours. Periactin is particularly effective for cholinergic urticaria, but is very sedating and stimulates appetite, resulting in weight gain. Hydroxyzine may have an advantage over diphenhydramine in some cases of urticaria and angioedema, and may be more effective as an antipruritic. Hydroxyzine is also effective as an antiemetic.

Side effects. In general, these are safe drugs. Side effects include sedation, which often decreases with continued use of the drug. Alcohol should be avoided while taking antihistamines. Patients may experience gastrointestinal side effects, including abdominal pain. The sedation effect may be an advantage, as in patients with severe pruritus, where

TABLE 14-9

NONSEDATING ANTIHISTAMINES ARE LISTED WITH THEIR SOURCE, TRADE NAME AND DOSE

Name	Derived From	Trade Name	Dose	Frequency
Fexofenadine	Terfenadine	Allegra	30 mg	bid
			60 mg	bid
			180 mg	Daily
Loratadine	Azatadine	Claritin	10 mg	Daily
			5 mg/5 mL	
Desloratadine	Loratadine	Clarinex	5 mg	Daily
Cetirizine	Hydroxyzine	Zyrtec	10 mg	Daily
			5 mg/5 mL	
Azelastine		Astelin	Nasal spray	bid

taking Atarax or Benadryl at night can reduce the itch and help the patient to sleep. Benadryl is the active ingredient of most OTC sleep aids.

Nonsedating Antihistamines

The drugs in this group are generally derivatives of sedating, first generation antihistamines. Table 14-9 presents preparations that are approved for use.

These drugs generally have a longer duration of action, from 12 to 24 hours. The response is individual, and the degree of sedation that occurs varies. Cetirizine has a higher frequency of sedation. Many are combined with decongestants, such as pseudoephedrine to increase effectiveness. However, some preparations have high concentrations of pseudoephedrine (240 mg in 24-hour preparations) that interfere with sleep. Some patients tolerate the drug by taking a combination that has a lower dose of pseudoephedrine (120 mg) and half the dose of antihistamine in the morning, and the other half of the antihistamine dose in the evening without pseudoephedrine.

Dual Acting Antihistamines

These drugs have an effect in directly inhibiting mast cells as well as blocking histamine. Others have a dual H1 and H2 effect (Table 14-10).

Patanol, Alomide, and Zaditor are useful in the treatment of allergic and vernal conjunctivitis. They exhibit an initial effect from the anti-H1 properties and a long-term effect from stabilizing mast cell membranes.

H2 Antagonists

These drugs have proved useful as adjunctive therapy to H1 blockers, especially in chronic urticaria.

Actions   Inhibit vasodilatation
           Block histamine feedback
           Block suppression of basophil chemotaxis
           Block histamine catabolism
           Enhance cell-mediated immunity
           Inhibition of gastric acid production
Examples   Burimamide
           Metiamide
           Cimetidine
           Ranitidine
           Oxmetidine

Decongestants

α Sympathetic agonists (e.g., pseudoephedrine)

Action

These drugs cause vasoconstriction. They are common adjuncts to antihistamines in commercial preparations.

TABLE 14-10

DUAL ACTING ANTIHISTAMINES

Preparation	Trade Name	H1 Effect	H2 Effect	Mast Cell Stabilizer
Azelastine	Astelin	++	ΔΔ	No
Olopatadine	Patanol	++	Weak	+++
Ketotifen	Zaditor	++	Weak	+++
Doxepin	Sinequan	++	ΔΔ	No
Iodoxamide	Alomide	++	Weak	+++

Note: This group of drugs has an effect in blocking H1 histamine receptors and in stabilizing mast cells. The + symbols represent the degree of the drug's effect.

Topical use is in common OTC preparations such as Afrin, Neosynephrine. Use of these preparations has the potential to cause rhinitis medicamentosa, which is hyperemia and mucosal hypertrophy in the nose. The condition results from repeated cycles for constriction and rebound dilation of blood vessels. Patients should limit topical use to no more than 2 days.

These drugs may be used for 2–3 days in the management of sinusitis to promote drainage.

Antileukotrienes

This is a group of drugs that specifically block the synthesis of an inflammatory mediator, or the receptor for the agent. The leukotrienes are synthesized by a number of inflammatory cells, including mast cells, macrophages, lymphocytes, polymorphonuclear cells, and eosinophils, using arachidonic acid as the substrate. Arachidonic acid is acted on by cyclooxygenase, which gives rise to prostaglandins or by lipoxygenase which initiates the leukotriene cascade. Leukotrienes cause bronchoconstriction, increased secretion of mucus and are chemoattractant for eosinophils, all major features of asthma. Inhibiting the leukotrienes is effective in about 65% of asthmatics.

The effect of these drugs may take 1–2 weeks to become apparent. The patient should be given the drug for 2 weeks to determine if it works.

This group of drugs is effective in treating asthma and allergic rhinitis. In rhinitis, antileukotrienes block the congestion and obstruction effects, since leukotrienes are nearly 5000-fold more potent than histamine at causing vasodilatation and transudation of fluid. These are the key mechanisms of chronic nasal congestion and bronchial mucosal swelling. The leukotrienes are also potent bronchoconstrictors.

LTD4 Receptor Antagonists

There are three active forms of leukotrienes, LTC4, LTD4, and LTE4 that have different properties. They all bind to the LTD4 receptor.

Montelukast

Brand: Singulair 4 mg (chewable tablet and sprinkle) 5 mg chewable tablet and 10 mg tablet

Indications: Asthma and allergic rhinitis

Dose: Once daily, preferably in the evening. No food restrictions

    1–2 years 4 mg sprinkle

    2–5 years 4 mg chewable tablet or sprinkle

    6–14 years 5 mg chewable tablet

    >14 years 10 mg tablets

Common side effects

- Headache
- Flu-like symptoms
- Cough
- Dizziness
- Rash, pruritis, urticaria
- Gastroenteritis
- Elevated liver enzymes

Zafirlukast

Brand: Accolate 20, 10 mg
Dose:

    7–12 years 10 mg bid
    >12 years 20 mg bid
    Must not be taken with meals or food (30 minutes before or 2 hours after meals)

Common side effects

- Headache
- Nausea
- Diarrhea
- Abdominal pain
- Fever
- Back pain
- Vomiting
- SGPT elevation
- Dyspepsia

Lipoxygenase Inhibitors

Zileuton. Zileuton blocks 5′lipoxygenase, thus effectively blocking all leukotriene synthesis. The disadvantage of this drug is that it requires qid dosing and is hepatoxic. There is no pediatric approval.

Brand: Zyflo
Dose: 600 mg qid
Side effects:

- Hepatoxic. Need to monitor liver function
- Abdominal pain
- Nausea
- Dyspepsia

Suggested Reading

Couriel, J. (2003). Asthma in adolescence. *Paediatr Respir Rev* **4**(1): 47–54.

Factor, P. (2003). Gene therapy for asthma. *Mol Ther* **7**(2): 148–52.

Federico, M. J. and A. H. Liu (2003). Overcoming childhood asthma disparities of the inner-city poor. *Pediatr Clin North Am* **50**(3): 655–75, vii.

Guevara, J. P., F. M. Wolf, et al. (2003). Effects of educational interventions for self management of asthma in children and adolescents: systematic review and meta-analysis. *BMJ* **326**(7402): 1308–9.

Lasley, M. V. (2003). New treatments for asthma. *Pediatr Rev* **24**(7): 222–32.

Lin, H. and T. B. Casale (2002). Treatment of allergic asthma. *Am J Med* **113**(Suppl. 9A): 8S–16S.

Payne, D. N. (2003). Nitric oxide in allergic airway inflammation. *Curr Opin Allergy Clin Immunol* **3**(2): 133–7.

Tarlo, S. M. and G. M. Liss (2003). Occupational asthma: an approach to diagnosis and management.[comment][erratum appears in CMAJ. 2003 Apr 15;168(8):966]. *CMAJ* **168**(7): 867–71.

Tokura, Y., M. Rocken, et al. (2001). What are the most promising strategies for the therapeutic immunomodulation of allergic diseases? *Exp Dermatol* **10**(2): 128–37; discussion 138–40.

Van Cauwenberge, P. (2002). Advances in allergy management. *Allergy* **57**(Suppl. 75): 29–36.

Wyrwich, K. W., H. S. Nelson, et al. (2003). Clinically important differences in health-related quality of life for patients with asthma: an expert consensus panel report.[comment]. *Ann Allergy Asthma Immunol* **91**(2): 148–53.

15

ENVIRONMENTAL CONTROL

Environmental control measures are an essential part of regulating indoor allergies by removing the allergen or providing a barrier between the patient and the allergen. The environment can be thought of as indoor and outdoor. Very little of the outdoor environment is available for the patient to control, and most of the measures that a patient can take involve avoidance of outdoor allergens and pollutants (Table 15-1).

INDOOR ENVIRONMENT

The factors that can aggravate allergies and asthma indoors can be considered as allergens and irritants.

Allergens

There are three main groups of indoor allergens: mold, insects, and animals.

Mold

There are a large number of molds that are found indoors, though many are outdoor molds that are brought indoors from outside. The most significant are *Aspergillus* sp., *Alternaria* sp., *Cladosporium*, and *Penicillium*, but any mold can become an allergen. The molds are found indoors in damp areas, such as leaky basements, under sinks and basins, behind damp walls, and in and around garbage. A major source of mold spores is the large reservoirs of carpets, upholstered furniture, bedding and heating and air conditioning ducts. Any source of standing water, such as humidifiers with a water pan, will also be a source of heavy mold contamination. Except for leaks and large concentrations of mold, most contamination is invisible.

Insects

The main indoor allergenic insects are house dust mites and cockroaches. Debris from other insects such as moths, flies, bugs, and beetles are less common causes of allergies, but are also contained in the complex mixture that is house dust.

House dust mites. Dust mites are microscopic, blind insects that live on shed skin and other sources of keratin. They require moisture and warmth and are critically dependent. They are usually found in mattresses, carpeting, and upholstered furniture. Feathers and foam are sources of the insect. The feces are the predominant allergen, but there may be reactions to the chitin in the body shell. The antigen is heavy and is not airborne to a

THE MAJOR GROUPS OF ENVIRONMENTAL AGENTS THAT CAN CAUSE AND AGGRAVATE ASTHMA AND ALLERGIC CONDITIONS

Allergens
  Mold
  Insects
      House dust mites
      Cockroaches
  Animals
      Domestic animals
  Pests
      Mice
      Rats

Irritants
  Tobacco
  Perfumes and scents
  Household cleaners
  Wood-burning fireplaces

Heating and Air Conditioning

Note: This is not an exhaustive list and is explained further in the text.

significant degree. Usually it becomes airborne briefly when the area is disturbed by walking on carpets or moving on a mattress.

Cockroaches. Cockroaches are mainly found behind walls and under floors and in drains. They are a major source of allergies in high-rise buildings, especially in areas with an indigent population. They usually seek food and water at night. It has been said that the ratio of visible to hidden cockroaches is as high as 1000:1. Like dust mites, they are a significant early factor in the development of asthma in young children.

Animals

Domestic animals. Cats and dogs are potentially highly allergenic. The shed antigen is light and easily airborne. It is found in saliva, urine, and on dander and hair. The animal licking itself may add to the level of antigen on the skin, but the antigen is

produced on the skin as well. In fact, it seems that the skin may be the primary source of the main antigens of dogs (Can f 1) and cats (Fel d 1). In general, more people seem to react to cat antigen than dog. Because the antigen is sticky, it is hard to remove from upholstered furniture, bedding and carpeting.

Pests. Mice and rats have potent antigenic proteins in dander and urine. They are emerging as a significant allergen in inner city areas. Mice may also be kept as pets. As with hamsters and other caged animals, there is very high mold and dust mite content in the cage.

Irritants

Tobacco

Smoking remains the most significant source of indoor irritants. Cigarette smoke can trigger acute asthma, increase the frequency of sinus disease, and is associated with a wide array of malignancies. There is mounting evidence that second hand smoke is equally dangerous, especially for children living with a smoker.

Perfumes and Scents

Strong perfumes, scented soaps, hair sprays, and air fresheners can trigger symptoms of allergic rhinitis or asthma.

Household Cleaners

Cleaners that contain bleach or ammonia are particularly irritating to the airways.

Wood-Burning Fireplaces

Wood does not burn completely, and there are byproducts of burning wood in a fireplace that are very irritating to the airways.

Heating and Air Conditioning

Forced air systems, which use ducts to carry warm or cool air, have more problems than radiators or baseboard heaters. The ducts collect dust, animal dander and mold, and blow them throughout the house.

INDOOR MEASURES

There are several key areas that should be considered.

- General measures
- Bedding
- Heating and cooling
- Room environment
- Animals
- Indoor irritants
- Floor coverings

General

Frequent cleaning is useful in reducing the level of dust and other allergens. Vacuum cleaners that incorporate a HEPA (high efficiency particle attractor) filter are more efficient at removing particles to sizes below 1 μm. Usual type vacuum cleaners incorporate bags that are inefficient filters and can blow about one-third of the dust that is picked up back into the atmosphere. The HEPA filter prevents this phenomenon. Furniture should be cleaned with a damp cloth so as not to brush more dust into the air. Dusters only throw dust into the air, and it settles elsewhere, giving the impression of cleaning. Blinds should be cleaned with a damp cloth. Hardwood floors and tile should be damp mopped or vacuumed.

Room Cleaners

Unlike HEPA filters in vacuum cleaners, room air purifiers with HEPA filters are not very useful. Most of the antigens that are present in the home are heavy, and do not remain in airborne suspension long enough to be cleared by the air purifier. Common examples are dust mites, mold and cockroach antigens. These heavy antigens settle quickly after being disturbed by walking or cleaning. However, the particulates of cigarette smoke and the danders of cats and dogs are exceptions which remain in air suspension and are cleared by the HEPA filter. For example, an antigen load of 40 ng/m of Fel d 1 (cat antigen) will induce asthma symptoms within 15 minutes in a sensitive individual who has asthma. This load can be reduced below 2 ng/m with a HEPA filter. In general,

though, the use of these filters has not been shown to affect the clinical outcome for asthma.

Furnace

This is also true of the furnace/air conditioning system. There are several filters on the market that are added to the furnace. These fall into two categories, electrostatic and HEPA. They will both remove particulates and other airborne particles. Installation should be accompanied by cleaning of the ducts. The same limitations apply to whole house filters as are found in room HEPA filters. Like the in room filters, they are useful for animal dander and other light antigens. The whole house filter is useful in situations where there is mold in the basement area that is carried to other parts of the house by the heating system. A good filtration system will prevent the spread of mold spores throughout the house. Whole house filtration systems are expensive, and the physician and patients should evaluate whether they will be useful in a particular situation. Window air conditioning units should be checked at the start of the summer and foam filters and pads should be replaced. The foam pads should be checked monthly during use.

Humidity

Humidification is a tricky issue in the home. Too low humidity will increase respiratory irritation and drying. There is an increased likelihood that the patient, especially a child may have epistaxis. On the other hand, too high humidity level (above 65%), will encourage the growth of mold and mites. A compromise range of humidity is between 35 and 45%, which will still provide comfort while minimizing the effect on mold and mite growth. Table top type vaporizers should be discouraged, and they produce water droplets, rather than humidity. In general, humidity is not visible. Particles of water that can be seen as a cloud or mist are large enough to carry mold spores, viruses and bacteria and increase the spread. The vaporizers also readily cause condensation, increasing the risk of mold growth. Furnace/whole house humidifiers should be of a continuous flow type, so that there is no standing water that will allow mold growth. The humidification pad should be changed at least once per season. These units have humidity level controls built in. For individual rooms, an evaporative type humidifier that has a foam pad or rotating drum and a fan that evaporates that water off the foam provides good humidification. A bacteriostatic should be added to the water, and the holding tray cleaned twice per week. These units usually hold a 2–3-day supply of water, so that there is a reminder to clean them. It is important that the unit have a humidistat so that the level of humidity can be controlled.

Bedroom

The use of throw rugs on bare floor is preferable to fitted carpet. Rugs can be picked up and it is easy to clean under them, which is not the case with fitted carpet. The backing of carpets is usually a foam material, and mites and mold grow readily in that environment.

Dust collecting books should be kept on shelves or out of the bedroom. They and the shelves should be regularly cleaned.

Clutter should be avoided. Clothing should be in closets that close, and laundry should be kept in a hamper with a lid. Children's toys need to be in a closet or toy box. Stuffed and soft, fluffy toys are prone to accumulate mites and mold. Since removing them is often traumatic for the child, they can be kept on a dusted shelf, but not in close contact on the bed. Washing soft toys and animals is recommended. Hot water should be used, and it is essential to ensure that the toy is thoroughly dry. Stuffed animals that have the appearance of being past their prime should be removed.

Other dust traps are drapes and blinds. The window coverings should be easy to clean, such as mini blinds. Heavy drapes are particularly hard to keep dust free and should be avoided.

The focus of the room is the bed, and this is where the patient spends a significant part of the day. The problem areas are the mattress and the pillows. Dust proof covers are the most useful method of keeping the dust contents, mites and mold, under control. These covers should be impermeable, yet be comfortable so that they do not interfere with sleep.

There are several brands of *mattress protector* available that are constructed in layers and fit tightly to the mattress and pillows so that they do not crackle with movement. The mattress protectors must be washed prior to first use, and it is important to follow the manufacturer's directions. Another problem with plastic on bedding is that it can be uncomfortable and hot. While well designed covers avoid this problem, the patients should be discouraged from placing a mattress pad on the protector, as the quilting will allow mites and mold to grow. The usual cost of a mattress protector is around $80, and pillow covers are $20. Ideally, the mattress and box spring should be covered. Because the protectors are expensive, patients can use a cheap plastic cover on the box spring. A key feature of these protectors is that they encase the mattress completely and zip closed. Some recommendations even include sealing the zipper with duct tape. Interesting, recent data have cast doubt on the clinical value of this practice, but for patients with allergies to mites and mold, these barriers remain a simple and useful means of avoiding the antigen. As always, recommendations should be tailored to the individual patient.

The pillows should be made of a hypoallergenic material, which is usually a polyester fiber. This type of filling material discourages the growth of mold and mites. On the other hand, feathers and foam contain spaces and pockets that hold moisture and allow mold and mites to flourish.

The comforter should also not contain feathers. Blankets should not be made of wool.

Bedding should be washed weekly in hot water at a temperature above 130°F to kill mites and reduce mold content. While fiber-fill pillows can be machine washed, it is difficult to ensure that they dry completely. They should be washed without the impermeable protectors.

A further problem area, especially for children, is the use of bunk beds. These space savers are large dust traps. The child who is on the top also is exposed to ceiling dust and allergens, while the child on the bottom is exposed to dust from the bed above, worsened every time the other child moves. If space allows, the beds should be separated.

One problem with these measures is that the patient, especially a child, may feel that their bedroom is stark and bare. This perception will discourage compliance. The essential aspect of environmental control in the bedroom is to reduce direct contact with the antigen. Bedding and pillows are prime examples of areas of close contact where a simple measure, covering the mattress and pillows, can have a large impact on the outcome. Other measures that are intuitive, like cleaning frequently, are also usually well tolerated. It is important that a patient understands the reasons behind environmental changes, or they are unlikely to happen.

Heating and Air Conditioning

Filters should be used on the central furnace and changed monthly. Radiators with hot water heat have the advantage of not blowing air across the room, but radiators are dirt and dust traps. They should be cleaned regularly and radiator covers are helpful in keeping the level of dust down.

Using filters on air vents is an effective way to reduce mite and mold laden dust from the heating system. Special precut filters are available, but are expensive. A solution that is as effective is to use rolls or sheets of the furnace filter material. These are available from hardware stores and are easily cut to size. The intake and return registers in each room can be removed, the filter placed behind it, and then the register is returned to the duct. These filters at the room level are more efficient than a central filter. They also have the advantage of helping to keep the level of dust accumulation in the ducts low following professional cleaning.

Animals

Animals are the most difficult source of antigen in the home. They not only have potent allergens that are released into the air, but also act as vectors to bring outdoor allergens into the house. The cat litter box is a rich source of mold. Another problem with domestic animals is that they are seldom actually confined to a particular area, and spread antigen throughout the house.

The obvious solution, to remove the animal from the home, usually meets with resistance from at least one family member. Even when the animal is removed, intensive cleaning is needed to eliminate the sticky antigen from furniture, carpets and drapes. It may take many months even after the animal is no longer in the home to reach acceptable levels of antigen.

General supportive measures should be used to remove reservoirs of animal dander. These include removing carpets, replacing drapes with mini blinds, and cleaning upholstered furniture. The most helpful measure is to wash the animal at least weekly. This reduces the antigen level while the animal is being washed. It was previously thought that there is a progressive reduction in the level of antigen that is produced even once washing was stopped. This is probably not true, and the animals continue to shed antigen once washing is stopped.

Allergy immunotherapy to dogs and cats may be indicated if the family will not remove the animal (see Immunotherapy for further details).

Other animals, particularly hamsters and rabbits, are popular. They have several problems from an allergenic point of view. The first is that they live in a cage, which is constantly soiled. This results in a high level of mold, which is also on their fur and can cause reactions when the animal is handled. There is also a high level of dust mites in the cage and the bedding material.

Farm animals tend to represent less of a problem, as they are more easily avoided. Reactions to indoor animals may be more severe because of more frequent exposure and the high levels of antigen in the home, where the patient spends much more time. Children are also more likely to play with domestic animals than farm animals.

Pests and Insects

Cockroaches are the most enduring pest, and are resistant to many pesticides. They are also highly allergenic. The usual method to deal with them is to spray with a strong insecticide. The problem with this approach is that the insecticides are very irritating and can aggravate asthma. If spraying is done, the patient should be out of the home for 6 hours following spraying. A preferable approach for asthmatics is to avoid potent chemicals that are powerful airway irritants. The use of boric acid powder along baseboards is effective in keeping the insects out of the room to some degree.

Cockroaches are very dependent on available food and water. Programs such as Safer Pest Control rely on this dependence to encourage the cockroaches to go elsewhere. The other advantage of this approach is that the families are placed in control of their environment, with a better chance that the gains made will be sustained in the long term. The essentials of this approach are to block access for the cockroaches to food and water. This is achieved by removing garbage, not leaving food on counters or tables, not leaving water in sinks and fixing leaks that would provide water. It is also important to fix cracks and caulk around pipes and cabinets. This approach has shown success in inner city housing where other measures have not succeeded. These measures are also helpful in reducing the occurrence of mold, since damp and garbage are major sources of this antigen.

The other group of pests that are pervasive and difficult to eradicate are rodents, usually mice, but also rats. The urine and dander of these animals have recently been shown to be highly allergenic. Measures to reduce available food and garbage are important for rodents as well as insects. Additionally, gaps to the outside should be closed using steel wool and caulking. Rodents are capable of squeezing themselves through the most unlikely looking spaces, so the attempt at closing these gaps must be thorough. Traps of various types are available. They will not be very successful unless the portals of entry are closed off, as animals will keep coming into the home.

Irritants

Tobacco

Smoking in the home should be strongly discouraged. Smokers should be encouraged to quit, and providing tobacco cessation information is useful. There are several excellent programs sponsored by the American Lung Association and the American College of Chest Physicians, for example, that can assist patients and parents to quit. It is important that people understand that the exposure of asthmatics to second hand smoke is likely to worsen the condition and cause acute episodes that could be life-threatening. An asthmatic patient who smokes is at risk for rapid deterioration of pulmonary function. If smoking continues, it should occur outside. Smoking in the car should be actively discouraged. A garage does not suffice, unless it is completely detached from the house and does not share a roof with the house.

Miscellaneous

Additional measures may be helpful in reducing the level of antigens.

Avoid the use of wood-burning fireplaces. Other sources of partial combustion, such as kerosene, should be used outdoors only.

If *gas stoves* are used, it is important to ensure that there is adequate ventilation.

Using a *fan in the bathroom* when showering to reduce condensation on the walls and other surfaces and decrease mold growth.

Removing outdoor footwear on entering the house to decrease the introduction of mold and other outdoor allergens into the house.

Using *nonirritating household cleaners*, especially avoiding bleach and ammonia.

The effectiveness of the use of antimite preparations is controversial. These are mostly tannic acid preparations, an example of which is Acarasan. While they may kill the mites, the products remain, including feces, and can still cause reactions. Whether the long-term use of these products results in reduction of mite load has not been clearly established.

School/Office

The patient usually has limited ability to reduce exposure at school or in the workplace. If exposure to a known allergen or irritant is not avoidable, the patient should take preventative medication doses. If the situation is a workplace setting, a protective mask may a be possible solution. If protective gear is part of normal use in the job, it is essential that the patient use the equipment. It is important for the employer to be aware of the situation and the risks to the employee, and a transfer to another position in the company or even another line of work may be the only solution.

The same issues apply to children in school. The school should be aware of the risks to the child. This is particularly true of classes where chemicals are used. Caution should be exercised in older schools where there may be mold and insects. Children allergic to animals should not be in classes where there are animals present.

OUTDOOR

The outdoor environment is not readily available for control by the patient. Some measures can reduce the impact on the patient.

Cold

Exposure to cold is a major trigger for asthma in adults and children. Children should avoid outdoor recess when air temperatures are below roughly 35°C. A scarf or ski mask should be worn to protect the airways from cold dry air. Patients should be aware that sudden changes in temperature, as in walking into a heated building from freezing, dry air can trigger an acute episode. They may need to use a bronchodilator dose immediately on changing temperature if this is a problem.

Exercise

Exercise is a common trigger for asthma. The more aerobic the activity, the more likely it is to cause serious symptoms. Patients should use prophylactic medication, which may include albuterol prior to activity, long-acting bronchodilators and controller medications (see chapter on Asthma).

CONCLUSIONS

The control of the environment is essential in a disease that is triggered by allergens and irritants in and around the home. Some suggestions follow:

Remove stuffed animals and other dust and mite traps.

Remove pets (washing has proven useful in reducing antigen load).

Use wood floors rather than carpets.

Replace air conditioning and heating filters frequently.

The use of air purifiers is of doubtful value.

Suggested Reading

Ahmed, D. D., S. C. Sobczak, et al. (2003). Occupational allergies caused by latex. *Immunol Allergy Clin North Am* **23**(2): 205–19.

Bhalla, P. L. (2003). Genetic engineering of pollen allergens for hayfever immunotherapy. *Expert Rev Vaccines* **2**(1): 75–84.

Boner, A., L. Pescollderungg, et al. (2002). The role of house dust mite elimination in the management of childhood asthma: an unresolved issue. *Allergy* **57**(Suppl. 74): 23–31.

de Blay, F. and E. Birba (2003). Controlling indoor allergens. *Curr Opin Allergy Clin Immunol* **3**(3): 165–8.

Eggleston, P. A. (2003). Environmental control for fungal allergen exposure. *Curr Allergy Asthma Rep* **3**(5): 424–9.

Golden, D. B. (2003). Stinging insect allergy. *Am Fam Physician* **67**(12): 2541–6.

Kurup, V. P. (2003). Fungal allergens. *Curr Allergy Asthma Rep* **3**(5): 416–23.

Sheikh, A. and B. Hurwitz (2003). House dust mite avoidance measures for perennial allergic rhinitis: a systematic review of efficacy. *Br J Gen Pract* **53**(489): 318–22.

Vance, G. H. and J. A. Holloway (2002). Early life exposure to dietary and inhalant allergens. *Pediatr Allergy Immunol* **13**(Suppl. 15): 14–8.

Weber, R. W. (2003). Patterns of pollen cross-allergenicity. *J Allergy Clin Immunol* **112**(2): 229–39; quiz 240.

16

ALLERGY IMMUNOTHERAPY

BACKGROUND

The concept of attempting to change the immune response away from an allergic reaction to a more conventional or nonallergic reaction dates back to the early part of the twentieth century. In 1911 Leonard Noon proposed a toxoid to prevent reactions to grass pollen. It was not until the latter half of the century that controlled studies demonstrated that allergy immunotherapy led to clinical improvement. Up to that point, most reports were anecdotal reports, and not scientific.

CLINICAL RESPONSES

A number of the immunologic changes induced by allergen immunotherapy have been reported to correlate with the clinical response. These responses include reduced sensitivity to the allergen on testing by titrated prick skin test, conjunctival and nasal challenge following immunotherapy. These findings correlate with a reduction of symptoms of rhinitis occurring during natural pollen exposure.

Early Reactions

There is a reduction in the immediate response to specific allergens in the eye and conjunctiva during the peak allergy season for that allergen. This response has been demonstrated in a number of clinical studies using a wide variety of indoor and outdoor antigens. The responses of patients were noted using a symptom score of nasal and ocular changes during the season for the allergen, or during a set period for perennial antigens. Patients receiving allergy immunotherapy demonstrated lower symptoms scores (high numbers indicate worse disease).

The response to immunotherapy (IT) has also been demonstrated by direct nasal or conjunctival challenge. There was a reduction in clinical response among patients and subjects who received immunotherapy. There is also a reduction in cell infiltrates and mediator release.

Bronchial responses have been measured using several criteria, including clinical score and cell and mediator release. Unlike the use in allergic rhinitis, there is controversy over the effectiveness of IT in asthma. Crude assessments, such as meta-analyses that encompass widely differing studies and techniques, seem to show an advantage. Carefully constructed, prospective, controlled studies are ambiguous, and do not show a clear advantage for IT. Patients with asthma should be carefully selected for IT to maximize the chance of success.

Allergy skin test may decrease rapidly following the initiation of IT. The clinical response with reduced symptoms is much slower. This suggests that there is a disconnection between clinical symptom improvement and allergy skin testing.

Late Reactions

There is reduction of the late cutaneous response following initiation of IT. In some studies, there is a greater reduction in the late cutaneous response than in the early. The late bronchial response is also reduced by IT.

MECHANISM OF ACTION

The principle behind allergy IT is inducing a class shift from the production of IgE to IgG in response to the allergen and to blunt the allergic response.

IgE initially increases, then decreases, and is ultimately much lower than the initial level. There is commonly a rise in serum IgE during the specific allergen season. This rise is blunted by allergy immunotherapy.

There is a change in IgG that has also been noted following the use of immunotherapy. There is an increase in blocking antibodies in the IgG1 and IgG4 subclasses, with a gradual shift to IgG4. There is considerable controversy regarding the significance of IgG4, which some authors have regarded as a reaginic antibody. The mechanism whereby this antibody can cause allergy is not clear. It is present in low concentration in serum, but specific IgG4 becomes predominant after 1 year of allergy immunotherapy. However, there is poor correlation between levels of blocking IgG1 and IgG4 antibody and clinical score. The levels of IgG4 are not reliable as a predictor of long-term outcome, and IgG4 levels may not be significant as a mechanism of action of immunotherapy.

Cell Effects

Basophils

Basophils have reduced release of histamine following in vitro allergen challenge with ragweed in patients undergoing ragweed immunotherapy. This is not a reliable response to measure the success of immunotherapy, and is more of a research than clinical tool.

Lymphocytes

Peripheral blood lymphocytes have a diminished proliferative response to ragweed following allergy immunotherapy with ragweed extract. This is an antigen specific response. There is also a reduction of IL-2. Decreased production of TNF-alpha has been seen following house dust mite immunotherapy. This response is thought to be due to the generation of suppressive T cells.

An increase in CD8+ T cells has also been observed following immunotherapy with house dust mite. There is a concomitant reduction in the number of infiltrating CD4+ T lymphocytes. However, there is an increase in the expression of activation markers MHC Class II antigens and IL2R following IT. There are some biopsy data that suggest that there is an increase of mRNA for IL2 and IFN-gamma. There was an inverse correlation between patients' seasonal symptoms and medication requirements during the pollen season and the number of cells expressing mRNA for IFN-gamma from biopsy samples.

IgE Receptor

Low-affinity IgE receptor (FcεRII) on B lymphocytes is increased following allergy immunotherapy, but this response seems to be antigen specific. The role of this change in surface receptors in altering the response to antigen is not clear.

Histamine Releasing Factor

Factors controlling the release of histamine by mast cells and basophils are altered by allergy immunotherapy. Unstimulated polymorphonuclear cells in culture discharge spontaneous histamine releasing factor (spHRF). This synthesis is further increased by the addition of a specific antigen to the culture which leads to the release of a second, antigen dependent type of HRF. The levels of both forms of HRF are reduced by allergy immunotherapy in an antigen specific manner, but some variation has been noted, depending on the antigen. It is likely that reducing or altering HRF reduces the response to an allergen following immunotherapy.

Blood Eosinophils

Immunotherapy alters the number and function of eosinophils. Asthmatic children receiving house dust mite immunotherapy had lower peripheral blood eosinophil counts than a group of house dust mite-sensitive children not receiving immunotherapy. Basophil counts among the group on immunotherapy are also reduced compared to levels in normal controls.

Topical levels of eosinophils are also decreased by allergy immunotherapy. This has been shown from nasal brushings in patients receiving maintenance ragweed therapy. The level of decrease in eosinophils correlated with the dose of ragweed antigen used in maintaining control. Allergen immunotherapy treatment for birch pollen–sensitive asthmatics prevented the seasonal rise in eosinophils in bronchoalveolar lavage (BAL) fluid, compared to control patients who did not receive immunotherapy. Eosinophil chemotactic activity was also suppressed by immunotherapy.

Mediator Release

Measuring serum eosinophil products, mainly cationic protein, revealed significantly lower values during pollen season in patients on IT than in controls who were not receiving therapy. There is normally a seasonal increase in eosinophil and neutrophil chemotactic activity in the serum and BAL fluid of sensitized patients. Several studies have demonstrated that immunotherapy blocks this seasonal increase to specific antigens, for example, house dust mite.

An inverse correlation has been noted between the response to immunotherapy and levels of serum platelet activating factor (PAF) in asthmatic children. There are also descriptions of reduction in IL-4 in serum following allergy immunotherapy, indicating a shift from Th2 to Th1 type immune response. A rise in gamma interferon and tumor necrosis factor has been described following specific allergy immunotherapy.

RATIONALE FOR INSTITUTING IT

Allergies impose a large burden on individuals and on the healthcare system.

There is a high level of utilization of health services by patients with allergic disease. Where quality of life assessments have been performed, they demonstrate significantly lowered scores in all domains of perceived quality. Even in allergic rhinitis, a disease generally perceived as trivial by those who do not suffer from it, there is significantly poor perception of the quality of life.

Missed school is a serious problem from atopic disease, and it has been estimated that allergic disease accounts for a total of nearly two million days lost per year. Children can suffer from behavioral problems and hearing and speech impairment. These problems have an impact on learning. For children with asthma, there are many consequences, including loss of school days, poor academic performance, inability to participate in sports and high utilization of medical services.

The parents of children and adults with allergic diseases miss work, accounting for a very large number of work days lost and lost income. They also use medical services to excess. One estimate places the direct and indirect costs for allergic rhinitis at $3.8 billion.

For many of these patients, conventional therapy is inadequate. For others, avoidance of triggering antigens is not feasible. These are patients who may benefit from IT.

INDICATIONS FOR IMMUNOTHERAPY

Immunotherapy is not a curative procedure, leading to, on average, 60% improvement in symptoms to specific antigens in responding patients. For this reason, careful selection is essential for a successful outcome. IT is a significant time and expense commitment on the part of the patient.

General Indications

There are differences in opinion regarding who should receive IT, and which patient will benefit. Suggested guidelines from the American Academy of Allergy, Asthma and Immunology include the following:

- A history that is suggestive of an allergic etiology for the patient's symptoms.
- Symptoms that correlate with exposure to the suspected antigen, for example the patient who has a positive test to ragweed should react in the fall in the northern part of America.
- The patient has poor control with conventional therapy.
- The patient is unable or unwilling to avoid the antigen, for example, a cat or a dog.
- The suspected allergy must be confirmed by allergy test by prick skin test or RAST.
- Before starting immunotherapy, intradermal skin test should be done to exclude other antigens.

Specific Indications

Allergic Rhinitis

Allergic rhinitis and allergic conjunctivitis are prime conditions for the use of allergy immunotherapy. They are usually well defined, symptoms are easily assessed and evaluated, and it is relatively easy to assess the effects of therapy. Moreover, these conditions lend themselves to environmental control measures.

Insect Sting Allergy

The stinging insects, bees, hornets, wasps, yellow jackets, and fire ants, can cause life-threatening reactions. In determining the need for allergy immunotherapy, it is important to assess the risk to the patient. The first distinction is whether the patient has had a systemic reaction. This involves distinguishing a large local reaction for disseminated responses.

- Large local reaction—The swelling is contiguous with the site of the sting without a break. This is not an IgE mediated reaction.
- Systemic reaction—there is swelling or rash discontinuously with the sting site. If the patient had any difficulty talking, swallowing or breathing, the reaction is automatically regarded as systemic.

The second distinction that needs to be made is whether the patient may have had anaphylaxis. The blood pressure is crucial in deciding whether the patient had a vagal response with a cold clammy appearance but maintained circulation and no shock or developed anaphylaxis with a fall in blood pressure. A history of anaphylaxis, difficulty breathing or swallowing is an absolute indication to consider IT.

Drug Allergy

Of the many drugs (see Urticaria) that can cause systemic reactions, only penicillin has been tested for immunotherapy. Even then the method used is not usual. Therapy for penicillin is a rapid or rush form of therapy. The result is a form of controlled anaphylaxis that is useful only in the acute situation. It does not confer a long-term benefit. Because this is a dangerous form of therapy, it is only used in patients who have severe infection where penicillin is the drug of choice. The patient should be monitored in an intensive care unit.

Asthma

There is considerable controversy regarding the use of IT in asthma. The best chance of success is in patients who have concomitant atopy. While some studies of IT in asthma have shown improvement in symptom scores in patients who have a strong allergic component, other sets of data show no improvement using the same parameters.

Physicians must make careful selection of patients for IT in asthma. As with allergic rhinitis, the greatest chance of success is in patients who have a well-defined allergic component. An example of an appropriate patient is one who has severe asthma in the fall that is difficult to control, and demonstrates ragweed allergy by history, and prick skin test. Since the primary management of asthma is by pharmacotherapy, failure of this modality should be a requirement for considering IT.

UNDOCUMENTED IMMUNOTHERAPY

Food Allergy

Allergic reactions to food are complex and can induce severe reactions, including anaphylaxis.

Since the route of entry is either contact or via the gastrointestinal tract, such allergies do not lend themselves readily to intervention by IT. There are very few studies in the literature on the use of IT for food allergy. The only route of administration of IT for food allergy, using peanut allergen—has been the oral route—has shown limited success. Administering food antigens by injection is far too dangerous for practical application. Currently, there is no evidence to suggest that the use of food antigens for IT is effective or safe.

Biting Insects

While stinging insects are a major cause of allergic reactions, biting insects generally only give rise to a local response. There is no evidence to suggest that IT has any success in treating this condition. For this reason, IT is not recommended for this indication.

Skin Conditions

Eczema. Atopic dermatitis is multifactorial condition. While allergies play a part in initiating pruritus in this group of diseases, the use of IT has proven ineffective in ameliorating this condition. There is no currently approved indication for the use of IT in eczema and other forms of atopic dermatitis.

Chronic urticaria. The etiology of chronic urticaria is only detected in about 10% of cases. Without understanding the source of the condition, it is unjustified to use a potentially dangerous intervention such as IT. Thus, there is currently no indication for use of IT to treat chronic urticaria.

ALLERGENS FOR IMMUNOTHERAPY

Preparation of Allergens

Example of allergens used in IT are listed in Table 16-1.

Crude Saline Extracts

Most allergens for therapy are prepared by extracting the antigen from an allergic source. For example, for aeroallergens, pollens of trees, grasses, and weeds are collected and suspended in saline.

TABLE 16-1

COMMON ALLERGENS USED FOR IMMUNOTHERAPY

Pollen
Trees
Grasses
Weeds
Mold
Alternaria
Aspergillus
Insects
Mites
Cockroach
Animal dander
Dog
Cat
Hymenoptera
Honey bee
Yellow jacket
Paper wasp
Hornets
Fire ants

Note: This is not an exhaustive list.

Following centrifugation, the supernatant fluid contains a crude extract of proteins that include the key allergenic component. Other simple extractions use the same process. The use of these extracts is limited by the relatively low concentration of major allergen present in the extract. As a result, they may not prove effective for IT.

Purified Extracts

Several methods have evolved to enhance the extraction of the major allergens present in pollen, animal dander, mold, and insects, including house dust mites. One such purified extract is that of ragweed, where the active antigen, antigen E, constitutes 6% of the total protein content in ragweed pollen. Because the percentage of antigen E protein is so low, the crude extraction process is much less effective than the purified process for IT. The active antigen has been determined for many substances using gel extraction and specific testing of subcomponents for their antigenicity. In the case of cat dander, the active antigen is a single protein termed Fel dI. There are numerous methods, both chemical and physical, used for bulk extraction of pure antigens.

Modified Allergens

Beyond purifying antigens, several investigators have attempted to increase their antigenicity and thus shorten the course of IT. Methods used include alum precipitation, haptenization (the addition of a highly antigenic molecule, for example, albumen, to the antigen, in order to evoke a greater immune response), and the development of allergoids, which are chemically modified or denatured allergens. Allergoids are safer to administer than unprocessed antigens because they stimulate an IgG response and carry a reduced risk of causing anaphylaxis. Some of the methods employed to enhance antigenicity and safety are shown on Table 16-2.

Nasal Administration

Several authors have examined alternative routes, such as nasal. An example is the use of grass pollen, where 32 patients in a double-blind controlled study showed reduced symptom scores and increased nasal threshold to allergen.

TABLE 16-2

MODIFIED ANTIGENS THAT ARE USED TO ENHANCE ANTIGENICITY

Alum precipitated
Alum-precipitated pyridine
Emulsified in oil
Formalin allergoids
Gluteraldehyde polymerized
IgE specific
Urea denaturation
PEG conjugated

Note: Some of the common methods under investigation are listed.

PATIENT SELECTION

History

A history suggestive of an allergic reaction is essential in considering IT. This history would include seasonal allergic rhinitis symptoms, seasonal allergic conjunctivitis, symptoms on exposure to animals, or symptoms in damp or musty environments. A patient history of food allergy, asthma where there is no atopic component, or atopic dermatitis, are not indications for IT. Patients with combinations of indicated and nonindicated conditions may still benefit from IT for the indicated uses only.

Specific Testing

The indicated history must be confirmed by specific allergy testing, using either in vivo or in vitro methods (see chapter on Investigation of Allergies). The pattern of allergy given in the history should match the seasonality of the allergen. For example, one should react to trees in the spring, grass in the summer, and weeds in the fall.

Failed Pharmacotherapy

The primary management of allergies and asthma is pharmacotherapy. IT should be reserved for those patients for whom medication proves ineffective.

Unavoidable Allergens

Another circumstance where IT may be indicated is in the situation where patients or parents cannot avoid an antigen. This would occur in the case of a domestic animal that the family does not wish to remove from the home. IT is a useful adjunct to other measures such as washing the animal and other environmental measures as described in Environmental Control.

Managing Concomitant Conditions

Many patients exhibit symptoms related to more than one allergy. Care must be taken to identify as many allergens as possible, and to manage the environment as well as is possible. For example, a child's reaction to pet dander may be exacerbated by a parent's use of tobacco in the home. Wood-burning fireplaces, strong perfumes, and household cleaners, are other examples of aggravating factors which can complicate a true allergy.

METHODS

The antigen is administered in increasing doses starting at a very dilute concentration, usually 1:200,000 w/v. A problem arises with most antigenic extracts. There is no consistent method of measuring the antigenic content, and thus dosage can vary greatly. Attempts are being made to standardize the measurement and concentration of allergens.

Initially, injections are administered weekly. The dose is given into the subcutaneous tissue of the upper arm. With all doses, patients must be observed for 30 minutes after the injection, because severe reactions will usually occur within that time period. It is important to note that a patient may develop a severe reaction at any point during the course of treatment, so the observation must occur after each dose. The greatest risk occurs during the first few months of therapy.

After each dose, the patient's response is measured by a wheal and flare at the site of injection. The dose is gradually increased weekly, based on the size of the wheal reaction. The goal of IT is to reach a maintenance dose, which the patient will receive for a total course of therapy of approximately 5 years.

SAFETY

There are several theoretical risks to this form of therapy. Patients may develop a severe allergic response, either locally at the site of injection or systemically. This reaction may include an aphy-laxis. A recent large study of 4578 patients spanning 162,436 injections, demonstrated reactions at the frequency of 1/1600 injections. The occurrence of these reactions correlated with the frequency of injection and season of injection. More severe reactions occurred early in the therapy rather than later.

As stated above, most severe reactions are observed within 30 minutes of the injection. Of described reactions, 73% were respiratory, and 76% were urticaria or angioedema. Seven percent of patients with reactions developed anaphylaxis. Local reactions include swelling and pain, while systemic reactions, in addition to those discussed above, include gastrointestinal effects and vaso-vagal responses.

Due to the risks of severe reactions, when administering IT, emergency equipment, as well as personnel skilled in recognition of reactions and CPR, must be immediately available.

UNPROVEN TECHNIQUES

Many methods are offered for elimination of allergic reactions. These methods do not show any advantage when subjected to scientific evaluation. Unproven treatments include provocation-neutralization, which is a method whereby a low concentration of antigen is placed under the tongue. This process supposedly reproduces the patient's symptoms. A second drop is then placed under the tongue, which "neutralizes" the reaction, relieving the patient's symptoms.

Another technique that has not been proven is measuring IgG precipitins in serum that are directed against food. It is claimed that these precipitins cause a variety of symptoms not traditionally associated with IgE mediated allergy. IgG is commonly produced in response to the ingestion of food, and may even be a mechanism that guards against food allergy. Double-blinded controlled cross-over studies do not support this method.

Suggested Reading

Beyer, K. (2003). Characterization of allergenic food proteins for improved diagnostic methods. *Curr Opin Allergy Clin Immunol* **3**(3): 189–97.

Canonica, G. W. and G. Passalacqua (2003). Noninjection routes for immunotherapy. *J Allergy Clin Immunol* **111**(3): 437–48; quiz 449.

Chung, K. F. (2002). Anti-IgE therapy of asthma. *Curr Opin Investig Drugs* **3**(8): 1157–60.

Golden, D. B. (2003). Stinging insect allergy. *Am Fam Physician* **67**(12): 2541–6.

Nelson, H. S. (2003). Advances in upper airway diseases and allergen immunotherapy. *J Allergy Clin Immunol* **111**(3 Suppl.): S793–8.

Prescott, S. L. and C. A. Jones (2002). An update of immunotherapy for specific allergies. *Curr Drug Targets Inflamm Allergy* **1**(1): 65–75.

Saltoun, C. A. (2002). Update on efficacy of allergen immunotherapy for allergic rhinitis and asthma. *Allergy Asthma Proc* **23**(6): 377–80.

Valenta, R. and D. Kraft (2002). From allergen structure to new forms of allergen-specific immunotherapy. *Curr Opin Immunol* **14**(6): 718–27.

Weber, R. W. (2003). Patterns of pollen cross-allergenicity. *J Allergy Clin Immunol* **112**(2): 229–39

INDEX

Page numbers followed by italic *f* or *t* denote figures or tables, respectively.